Broken Whole

A California Tale of Craziness, Creativity and Chaos

Keith Adams

chipmunkapublishing
the mental health publisher

All rights reserved, no part of this publication may be reproduced by any means, electronic, mechanical photocopying, documentary, film or in any other format without prior written permission of the publisher.

>Published by
>Chipmunkapublishing
>PO Box 6872
>Brentwood
>Essex CM13 1ZT
>United Kingdom

http://www.chipmunkapublishing.com

Copyright © Keith Adams 2010

Edited by Aleks Lech

Chipmunkapublishing gratefully acknowledge the support of Arts Council England.

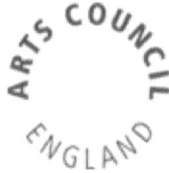

Broken Whole

To Ben

Keith Adams

Broken Whole

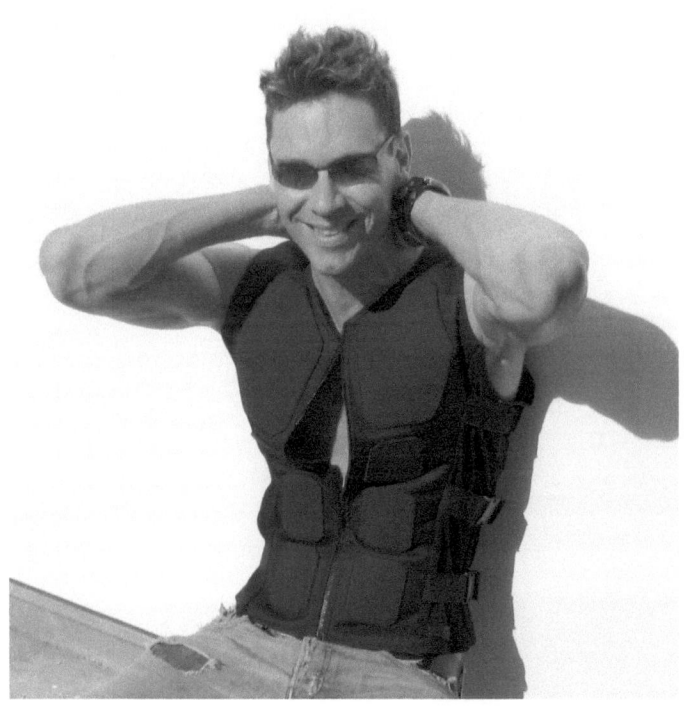

Keith Adams

Author's Note

All of the events in this book are true, although I predict that at times you may find them hard to believe. In these scandal-mongering, Freysian days, I do want to protect myself from claims of *making things up*. Many of the things that happened were recorded almost in real time on my blog, *brokenwholeblog.blogspot.com*, which has been online since early September of 2007, just a couple of weeks after some of the particularly colourful episodes, and I'd be happy to provide corroboration from medical and other records, upon request.

If you compare timelines and details between this book and my blog, however, you'll see a few very minor discrepancies, made for the sake of better pacing. I rewrote a couple of blog entries as integral parts of chapters, and transmuted one blog entry into conversation. Additionally, in the chapter which takes place in Dallas, I excluded any details about the work I was doing there, for obvious reasons: I still work as a senior developer for the same large software company as I did before and during the crisis.

I also changed the names of a couple of people who requested it. And, finally, I invented a surname (but not the actions or situation) of an officer in the chapter describing my being jailed by the LAPD. The officer in question, in the unlikely event he should ever read the book, will undoubtedly know that I'm talking about him.

On a separate note, since my publisher is British, they, of course "corrected" my Americanized spellings and grammar to the point where the prose frequently reads strangely, even to myself. I can only assure you that in British English it's apparently correct to say "I had got" instead of "I had gotten."

A Prelude to Insanity
Hollywood Boulevard, Hollywood, California, August 11th, 2006

I have always been strongly compelled to organize, categorize and understand every piece of information in my life. Now, as I felt my mind expanding infinitely in all directions, the flood of ideas through my brain was becoming almost impossible to handle. I was, for the moment, still able to control it, but I was close to being overmastered. The hardest thing was to figure out simple priorities against the raging background of my thoughts. And now the pressure was vastly increased by the screamingly high priority of not worrying my partner, Ben. He'd called me, out-of-the-blue, almost in tears because I was late for our meeting with our couples' counsellor, and I'd immediately set off to try to get across to West Hollywood.

At all costs, I thought, I had to protect him from worry. For weeks, I'd known that my increasingly confident and ambitious demeanor had made Ben anxious. I knew he thought that I was becoming slightly manic, so I'd got into the habit of concealing things from him: I didn't want his worry to restrain me from achieving my goals. Ben's last boyfriend had had episodes of intense mania as well, so this only increased my desire to hide from him all signs of any behaviour that he might wrongly interpret as manic.

For the moment, I could still wrestle my thoughts to a stand-still long enough to remind myself, every other minute, that it wasn't life-or-death. If I missed the meeting with our counsellor, Ben would be upset; very upset: but we'd get through it.

At the Renaissance Hotel on Highland, I tried to get a taxi, but the hotel staff ignored me. I became briefly and savagely furious with them until, once again, I managed to recall that my sense of urgency was self-imposed. But that thread of rational thought kept disappearing in the vastness; I couldn't hold onto it for more than a few seconds at a time. Each time it slipped my grasp, my focus would return to the urgency of protecting Ben at all costs.

I wasn't scared about myself, however, until I rounded the corner onto Hollywood Boulevard. And then I felt, just for a second, that it might be possible to drown in the deluge of my own thoughts.

I tried again to hail a cab. It was rush-hour; traffic barely moved, and all the cabs were full. I was, by now, almost panicking with the urgency of saving Ben. It had finally become impossible for me to have a rational perspective; I really was drowning.

I redoubled my pace, crossing through traffic to catch a cab in the other direction, anything. Once more I momentarily recalled the lack of real urgency, but only briefly, before crashing back, with increased violence, into a skewed sense that making the meeting with Ben and our couples' counsellor was life-or-death.

I steeled myself: 'Calm down, there's no rush.' A second later, I looked at the time, and started to run. The clash of priorities began to feel like a pile driver in my head; then a constant thunder. I ripped my expensive watch – a sexy, masculine watch with a wide leather strap that Ben had given me – off my wrist, and threw it, along with my cell-phone, into a parking lot, hoping that if I could no longer tell the time, the raging confusion would cease. But it only got worse.

Dimly through the clattering chaos, I momentarily heard a shining clear note: instead of worrying about Ben, I should take care of myself. This was my own crisis now, not Ben's: I was falling headlong into the void, and had to save myself. Moreover in saving myself, I'd save Ben too. If I lost my mind, Ben would shed far more than the few tears he'd cry at my missing our counselling appointment. It seems so obvious now; but that's a symptom of mania: that you can get so consumed by something that it makes you blind to all other priorities. In this case I was so driven to protect Ben that I was quite literally driving myself insane.

That gleaming note I'd felt moments earlier disappeared again in the gathering murk; I felt my sanity slipping away; I knew I needed to medicate myself immediately, either with drugs or alcohol. I pitched into a Mexican restaurant.

'I need a drink,' I grated out to the petite hostess, who looked at me worriedly, taking in the contrast between my wannabe-superstar appearance – six-foot-six, hair spiked with blond highlights, dressed in a tight-fitting, black open-necked Miu-Miu shirt – and the desperation presumably written on my features.

'You'll have to wait for a table.'

'You don't understand, this is an emergency,' I shouted.

She looked at me as if I were an alien, and then shrugged. I strode into the bar, grabbed a bottle of tequila, and walked out, ignoring the bartender's flailing arms and angry shouts.

I was on Sunset Boulevard by now, just east of La Brea. I drank about a fifth of the bottle: it tasted foul. Vodka is my drink, I thought randomly. My mind was still falling into chaos; the alcohol wasn't working.

I went into a 7-Eleven, where the cashier looked up at me, startled, seeing the open bottle of tequila in my hands, not exactly looking like a typical wino.

'Call 911!' I said, urgently.

The cashier barely even made eye-contact with me before switching back to his customer. I couldn't understand why nobody could see my pain. I was running into intense alienation wherever I turned.

I shouted at him, 'Call an ambulance, now!'

'Fuck off!' he told me.

I was amazed that he didn't seem the least bit scared of me. I slammed my fist onto the counter, and poured the bottle of tequila all over it.

Broken Whole

'Now will you call the fucking police?' I needed help, any kind of help. I knew I needed to be restrained and medicated.

A young gay customer yelled at the cashier, 'Call 911!' The kid led me outside.

'Here, I'll call them,' he said, soothingly.

I tried to sit down, but I couldn't keep still. He couldn't get through to 911; he was on hold for ten agonizing minutes; I couldn't wait. I crossed the street through moving traffic, and entered the strip-mall on the corner, which contained a Starbucks, nail salons, and some jewellery stores. I thought the police would come eventually, and I was concerned now that they'd think me dangerous, that bullets might fly.

The tequila was finally slowing down my thoughts. Somehow, I suddenly instinctively knew the worst of the crisis was passed; I'd saved myself. But there were still the consequences of my actions to deal with, and I was still far from being myself. I heard sirens, so I went into one of the salons to sit peaceably, my hands clearly visible so the police could see I wasn't armed (although it's not clear why I thought there was the possibility of a shoot-out). I was completely exhausted and intolerably thirsty. The tall Asian transsexual who was doing somebody's nails, kept looking over at me, a half-smile alternating on her pretty face with curiosity. I prayed she wouldn't say anything to me.

The police never came, so eventually I went outside. I still wanted to go to the emergency room, but maybe now I could do it without police involvement, I thought. I convinced a kindly Filipino security guard that I was having a medical crisis, and he lent me his cell-phone so that I could call 911.

He had, ironically, a blue-tooth headset, my first exposure to one despite my recent over-immersion in technology, and it took me a while to get it to work for me. But I couldn't get through to 911 - I was kept on hold for even longer than the kid across the street had been. I knew Ben would be worried. It seemed impossible, but it had only been thirty minutes since I had left the Renaissance after failing to get a taxi there.

I finally gave up on getting through to 911, but I didn't know who else to call. I didn't want Ben to know what had happened - at least not yet. But Ben's cell-phone number was the only number I knew by heart, and neither of my therapists had listed phone numbers, so finally I had no alternative but to call Ben. He was frantic. He'd been calling and calling, getting my voicemail. I told him my cell-phone was dead, and asked him not to ask me any questions; just come and pick me up.

At last I could let the tension breathe out of me. I thanked the security guard for the use of his phone and asked him if he could please find me some water. He looked at me dubiously, so I started to pull off my $300 belt to offer in exchange for a bottle of water. He relented and got me a bottle of water, declining the belt.

When Ben picked me up, I had to figure out how to explain to him everything that had happened that day (because, you see, this headlong rush through Hollywood was only the climax of an astonishing day.) I knew it wasn't the right time to tell him anything about what had preceded his tearful call from our counsellor's office less than an hour earlier. Nonetheless, my mind was still racing, and there was the manic temptation to explain myself fully. I kept holding onto the fact that I couldn't possibly tell him everything without scaring him; I had to simplify things. I kept saying to myself 'breathe', as a mantra to remind myself, through the haze of explanations yearning to be spoken, not to be driven to make Ben understand everything. I wrote 'breathe' on a scrap of paper as we drove home, because I didn't trust myself. And once I got home, I wrote it out again, on more scraps of paper, so I'd see it everywhere.

Later that night, as I got ready to take a shower, I looked at the scrap of paper on the sink with the word 'breathe' written on it. I suddenly had the image of Ben

Broken Whole

finding it, picking it up, and thinking it was another indication that I was not entirely in my right mind. We had a decorative bowl in the living-room full of pebbles of green glass bought from Pottery Barn. So after my shower, I grabbed a few green pebbles, and left them in inconspicuous places replacing the pieces of paper (they being so much less obvious than tiny bits of paper, of course.) Now I knew that every time I'd see one of those pebbles, it would remind me of 'breathe', and I'd stop trying to put into words what was going on in my racing mind.

But would I still remember 'breathe' in the morning? I surreptitiously stuffed a pebble underneath the sheet on my side of the bed, knowing that whenever I woke up, the physical discomfort would reconnect me to 'breathe'.

The next morning, things returned to a surprising degree of normality between us. We were both anxious about what had happened, but also eager to please each other. I felt sure that I'd never again let worry for Ben drive me to the edge of insanity. I also knew that it was going to take a lot of dialogue before he could fully understand what had happened the previous day. I had no idea there were even worse days to come; that the first, as yet undiagnosed, manic episode of my life hadn't wrought, by any means, all the damage it held in store.

Book I – The Story So Far
A Brief History of a Person

What is a person? How do you become the person you are? What is the real you, anyway? Do these questions sound familiar? Being hopelessly introspective, these are questions I've asked myself many times. But I never expected them to become as central to my life as they did in the summer of 2006. How did a small-town, working class boy from north-east England end up being that guy careening through Hollywood, one day, at the age of forty-one, on the verge of truly losing his mind? It certainly didn't happen overnight, although it seemed that way at the time. It was the inevitable culmination of four decades shaped by experiences, large and small.

Somewhere around the age of seven, my nature abruptly changed ... for the worse. In before and after snapshots in my mind's eye, I can see both versions. It's the beginning of the summer vacation, and I'm leaving kindergarten for the last time, on a golden June afternoon. Laughing and joking with my friends, I somehow see a bunch of girls clustered around the school-gate, all bemoaning my departure. While I'm quite sure that wasn't actually the case, I vividly remember how at home with myself I was - a happy-go-lucky, well-adjusted kid, excited about the future, full of promise, mind already secretly set on a future as a famous scientist.(I had, by this time, got over an obsession, shared with my brother, Neil, about being a bus driver.)

Six weeks later, I'm shivering on the floor of the assembly hall in Mowbray Road Junior School, not from the cold – although along the coast of north-east England it's not unknown for the temperature to dip into the fifties in the daytime even during the summer – but with anxiety, loneliness, and an acute sense of inner and outer ugliness. It marked the beginning of four years of misery, during which I had few friends, and began to see myself as *other than*.

For most of my adult life I've wondered about what happened during those six weeks to change me so much, but have never come to an explanation that feels like the truth. I have the strong feeling that if I hadn't endured those four solitary years at Mowbray Road, I'd have never known the ailments of adulthood that would deeply damage my psyche. I'd have steered a different path, less cautious, carried along by the feeling I could do anything I set my mind to. I might have been a golden boy. Maybe I'd have gone to Cambridge, and got a first in astrophysics, after which I'd have been snapped up by Cal Tech in Pasadena to become a pioneer of string-theory (which was hatching around the time I went to college, where I did indeed study physics and astronomy). I'd have been invited onto my favourite BBC television show, the science program *Horizon*, and, wearing a tweed jacket, thick, black-rimmed national health glasses, and an eccentric hat, and, I'd endeavour to make high-energy physics understandable to the masses, while gesturing with the unlit pipe in my hand.

You're probably thinking that since it sounds like few of those wonderful things happened, I must be a depressed loser, so why should you read this book? To begin with I claim not to be a loser – I'm a successful, robustly healthy, well-paid software-developer, living with a smart, sexy boyfriend – a professor at UCLA – in our house in the Hollywood Hills, with two dogs running around in the den. At the risk of adding to the belief, now suddenly dawning in your mind, that I may not be a loser, but might be rather full of myself, I have to announce that I'm "told" I'm good looking. Damn it, I hate that phrase. You're trying to have your cake and eat it, boasting simultaneously of your modesty and your looks. I *am* good looking. It's taken me years to accept this, and the struggle with body-image is a major strand in this story, but it would be disingenuous to deny it, since my height and physical presence are important to the story. And I'm not even lonely – far from it, I have an abundance of friends both here in Los Angeles, and in San Francisco, where I lived for twelve years before I moved to LA to live with Ben, my partner for life – a life that is fine, by any standard.

As you might expect, having read the prelude to this memoir, there was a ... blip ... somewhere on the road to my present stasis. Well, more than a blip, actually ... more like a supernova, collapsing into a black hole. Over a few blazing months, in 2006, everything that I'd experienced, all the strands of my life, wove together into a singularity, and I became fully realized, whole and complete. Finally, it really did seem like I could do anything I wanted. I believed I was about to become a sort of epochal intellectual / spiritual guru / gay Hollywood superhero / celebrity-messiah all rolled into one. (And you thought I was conceited before!) I couldn't have imagined how wrong I was, and that there was going to be a serious of increasingly dangerous crises just ahead of me, culminating in the longest night of hell in my life.

In the same way that all of my life story fed into what happened in 2006, some set of events or experiences changed me as a seven-year-old, and I've spent many hours in therapy (I feel your groan) trying to figure out what it was. The most obvious candidate was a tiny little incident that happened with my dad, an incident which was seemingly innocuous and inconsequential, at least to my dad, who has no idea how his offhand comment almost ruined my life.

To demonstrate how large this incident looms in my psyche, I can describe the time when I first told the story out loud. I was a tall, skinny, gawky graduate student in Philadelphia, pursuing a PhD in alternative energy. (My quest to be an astrophysicist had unfortunately been derailed by a misguided dalliance with fundamental Christianity. I somehow believed that "God" wanted me to do something socially relevant with my life. I blame my career misdirection on him.)

I was out of the closet by this time, but helplessly inexperienced and naïve both in love and emotion. I didn't remember when I'd last cried. Years of concealing my homosexuality, and the belief, instilled through being raised in the macho culture of north-east England, that emotions are effeminate, had buried my true personality under layers of self-consciousness.

The strange thing is that although I wanted to connect, I also pushed people away. I seemed to look for confrontation. I allowed myself to get bent out of shape whenever somebody asked my height. (People – complete strangers – feel it's perfectly fine to, out of the blue, in an elevator full of other strangers, turn to you and say, with earth shattering originality, and a note of incredulity in their voice, 'How tall are you?' I always want to respond 'How long have you had that carbuncle on your nose?') I remember one time I was in a bathroom stall in a gay bar in Philadelphia. I hate American bathroom stalls to begin with, since everybody else all but sees everything, particularly if the person in the stall is six foot six. This time, I was peeing, and some kid had the nerve to ask me my height over the partition, while I was peeing. I told him 'Fuck off you stupid queen.'

Despite my touchy relationship with the world, and, specifically, people, it's not as if I was socially backward – indeed, I had a lot of friends, both in school and out. But I was shy, and dry. And I yearned to cry. I know that sounds a bit precious, but since it's accurate, I'll leave it standing.

I spent one tortured, rainy Thanksgiving weekend, alone with nothing but the company of my tuna melts, in my apartment above the Pleasure Chest, in Center City, Philadelphia. This was in the late eighties. Ricardo, my cute Mexican roommate, a gentle souled, culturally sophisticated PhD music composer at Penn whom I fairly worshipped, was away with his awful Scandinavian girlfriend. I should take that back – her "awfulness" consisted entirely of the fact that she was Ricardo's girlfriend, which is hardly her fault. When she wasn't around, Ricardo and I would spend hours talking about music, film, philosophy, history. When she was there, in contrast, I'd just hear them banging each other in the room next to mine.

I fairly yearned to have emotions, and watched *Ordinary People* three times that weekend, hoping that I'd cry. Not only did I have the most tremendous crush on Conrad Jarrett, the young protagonist, but I envied him that great scene with Judd Hirsch where he finally cries, sweeping things off shelves. It reminds me now of some of my own therapy sessions – that is apart from the crying, and the sweeping things off shelves.

If I couldn't cry watching Conrad, then maybe I could become Conrad. I had the idea that acting lessons might unlock my heart. The Wilma Theater was just round the corner, offering low-priced classes with Gordon Phillips (of the "Gordon Phillips Method" – maybe you've heard of it?). Phillips was a lascivious, grey-bearded, dirty old man. Since the object of the class – as with all method acting – was to emote, it offered him the chance to be emotionally intimate with cute young women, and offered the young women the opportunity to emote without having to pay for more expensive talk-therapy. We guys were lucky to get a quick half-hour of attention.

The entire first series of ten classes was devoted to each of us doing a single monologue. The idea was that you'd learn the words of the monologue without punctuation or meaning, that is, just as a series of words. Then, in class, you'd be asked to recall something from your life that brought forward the appropriate emotion for the monologue. Phillips would lead you through your memories, while you sat with your eyes closed, perhaps holding Phillips' hand (if you were a girl), and just when you touched the core of the emotion, he'd tell you to speak the monologue.

I didn't really think it would work with me – I was far too self-conscious and controlled. Looking back, I'm amazed I even put myself in that situation given how averse I am to being emotionally manipulated. Perhaps that aversion is something I've developed since then, and back then I was more malleable. But there was an even greater problem – I felt I had no strong emotional experiences on which to draw. Nothing had ever happened to me, I felt, so deeply buried were my softer sensibilities by now.

It wasn't that I was, by nature, an unemotional person – in fact, quite the reverse. One of my strongest memories from childhood was the day upon which my dad, my brother Neil and I were taking a day-trip to Edinburgh; I looked back into the kitchen to see my mother's arms elbow deep in the non-automatic washing tub. The thought of us enjoying Edinburgh while my mother slaved away at home filled me with sorrow, and I ran upstairs to my bedroom to hide my crying from my dad.

But I was raised in a very macho, working-class culture, which my dad exemplified, and any tender impulses were squashed by derision, criticism, or, at best, a look on the face that I know only too well how to interpret. For instance, I was getting ready, when I was a mid-teen, to go to Newcastle, the nearest big city, to see *On Golden Pond*, starring Katherine Hepburn and the Fondas, Jane and Henry. My dad put me down with 'Why do you want to see a girl flick?' So, since I worshipped my dad, I gradually learned to bury those things that didn't fit with his image of a healthy boy. I was a quick study, and learned these lessons well. I didn't know I was doing this. It only became apparent to me much later in life, when I wondered what had happened to the empathy that was second nature to me as a kid.

In any event, when it came to choosing an emotional event as the basis for my monologue in acting class, I drew a blank. *Now*, I can think of lots of things I could have used from my earlier life, most of them centred on my body-image. When I was a teenager, my parents didn't have enough money to buy clothes that kept up with my rapidly extending limbs. And besides, I was already tall for my age, not to mention broad-shouldered. Clothes just didn't fit: my sleeves and trouser legs were always too short. For my socks not to show, I'd have to unfasten the button of my pants, slip them lower than my waist, tighten the belt, and pray. We'd buy my clothes in the adult department, and I'd cringe when my mother would screech 'Eeeh, he's only fourteen, you know!'

I was fully proportional, and while I'm not one to brag about my anatomy, I will admit that my feet were rather large. It was unfortunate that we came from a ship-building town, since it gave people license to say things like 'Did you get those boots at Swan-Hunters (one of the local shipyards)?' Even worse, I was cursed with the last name 'Adams'. 'Doo-doo-doo-doo. Click. Click. Doo-doo-doo-doo. Click click.' The beginning of the theme tune for the *Addams Family* will always stick in my craw. They called me Lurch, of course. Kids would laugh at me from across the street, and shout mean things. My walk to school became a mad, secretive dash to avoid humiliation, roving far afield from a direct route in order to avoid school kids. My body became a curse to me, and I moved lock, stock and barrel into my head.

All of this should have provided plenty of fodder for tears of reminiscence, but in fact the only thing I could come up with was the tiny little incident with my dad. So that's where we started when it was my turn to do the monologue.

> Phillips: *'Close your eyes, Keith, and think back to when you were that seven-year-old. Where are you?'*
>
> Adams: *'I'm in the living room of our house. My aunty Olive is here, smoking with my mom, and I'm horsing around with my dad.'*
>
> Phillips: *'Describe the room; let your mind go back there.'*
>
> Adams: *'The carpet looks like it belongs in a multiplex ...'*
>
> Phillips: *'Describe it like you would have done as a small boy.'*

Broken Whole

Adams: *'I love swirling my finger around the patterns in the carpet. The room is full of cigarette smoke. I'm bored. How can they talk so much?'*

Phillips: *'What's happening now, Keith?'*

Adams: *'My dad is grabbing my wrists with one hand. He's pushing his glasses up his nose.'*

Phillips: *'Does he say anything?'*
Adams: *'He says ...'*

And then, to my utter astonishment, I sob. *'He says I never knew you had such skinny wrists.'*

The monologue that followed was a blur. Afterwards I felt raw and bruised, and almost angry at Phillips for exposing me. I'd gotten what I'd wanted, though. I'd cried.

Years later, in therapy, looking back both on the original incident and the acting class, I wondered if the incident with my wrists was responsible for the change in my nature during those six weeks between schools. I do know it had a powerful effect on me that stayed with me even through my late thirties, albeit in an increasingly less virulent form. At the time, I ran upstairs and looked at my wrists in the mirror, and saw to my horror that they looked nothing like my dad's. They were thin and delicate. In fact, when I came to think of it, my arms were skinny too, and I suddenly noticed, after I took my shirt off, the bony knobs of my collar bones sticking out beneath my neck, and the ribs down my flank, which you could count. How could I never have noticed this?

Although I don't think this, in itself, was enough to cause the wholesale change in my personality apparent when I started my new school, certainly over the course of years I grew to detest my body, and concealed it underneath thick sweaters, even in summer. The only time I remember crying as a teenager was when my mother asked me why I didn't take my sweater off if I was so warm, and I sobbed, as I told her I was too skinny. Swimming class in high school was a never-ending nightmare, and it wasn't until college that I had the courage to wear a short-sleeved shirt – a button-up blue-striped cotton shirt (I wasn't yet gay enough to know that tall guys shouldn't wear stripes.) I wore that shirt all through my last summer as a student in London, waiting for my exam grades. I even began to think I wasn't completely unattractive. I had good proportions, broad shoulders, and high cheekbones, and wide blue-green eyes topped by long eye lashes. (People used to say I had beautiful eyes. In fact, that's the only compliment I used to get. I wonder if something happened to my eyes, because it's been years since I heard that compliment.)

I was wearing that same striped shirt on the day I arrived on campus, abroad for the first time in my life, at the University of Pennsylvania, to register for classes for my PhD course. It was blisteringly hot and humid, and I was the only person not wearing shorts.

On campus, I was immediately agog at the beauty of the American undergrads. There was an eighteen year old wearing a sleeveless t-shirt, the sides torn half way open to reveal, behind his rounded biceps, the edges of a muscular chest. Everywhere, blithely care-free kids seemed entirely at home in their bodies, completely unaware of any self-consciousness. I went back to my room and stared at myself in the mirror, hating the bony death-head's skull (that was the exact term I wrote down in my journal) atop a stick-like body, and the skeletal bones poking out of the short sleeves of that blue striped shirt I'd foolishly thought flattering.

It seemed, back then, impossible that I should ever learn to be at peace with my body. But, like so many gay boys, I would blossom with time – a lot of time. I began to work out, and, by the time I was twenty-seven, when I moved to San Francisco bearing a newly minted new green-card, I had reasonable musculature clad on my still skinny bones. (To put thing in perspective, even at this stage, after several years of working out, my 6'6 frame filled out at 175 lbs.) I was experienced in romance by now, and had fallen in love with a beautiful black man named Shaun, and had then forcibly broken my heart after realizing he loved me but didn't *love* me. But it wasn't until I started to receive treatment for the chronic fatigue syndrome that came on me in my mid twenties, that I understood that there was actually a reason why I'd always been so skinny: I was way short on testosterone (and that insufficiency was one of the prime movers behind my fatigue). After starting up on testosterone replacement therapy, I finally began to build the sort of body that could put to rest the demons of childhood. Or at least tell them to lie down and be fairly quiet.

So it is no longer surprising to me, perhaps, but still quite ironic, that during the after-glow of my blazing streak across the Los Angeles landscape in 2006 – the events to be related through the main body of this book – I did something people had been asking me about for years, and took myself to a modelling agency, one of the most prominent in the U.S., if not the world. I'll not play coy by refraining from telling you the outcome: I didn't get accepted. But, astonishingly, while sitting at lunch directly after the failure at the modelling agency – feeling not at all cowed by rejection, so strong did my self-confidence remain - all of the pieces fell into place with a resounding clink, and I finally, in a piercing moment of manic insight, figured out why I'd changed so much at the age of seven. And to find the answer to that, I'm afraid you *will* have to read the rest of the book.

Being Here

So what is it, after all, that defines who you are? A lot of people never ask themselves this question, particularly here in the United States, this country of extroverts, where few people are introspective enough to dig into their psyche. By my early forties I was living with the new love of my live, Ben, in our house in Hollywood. Although depression rumbled here and there in the background, I was beginning to believe that I too had found myself. Yet sometime in 2006, that question became open again. I began what I thought was a permanent recovery from depression, and thought I was finally becoming what I'd secretly always supposed I would be: somebody rather magnificent, the golden boy with the faculties of a wise, experienced man.

Depression is not interesting to read about at length. But as much as I yearn to immediately launch into the violently colourful events that spawned this book, it would be impossible for anyone to place those events in context without understanding the completely contrasting grey murk that both preceded the violent hues and, in part, precipitated them. But before delving into the muddy waters of depression, it might be timely to recount the origins of this book - very briefly, for that will give you a taste of "my forty-first year" (the original name of this book), and illustrate why the accelerated growth I experienced in the late summer of 2006 was so infinitely appealing to me.

Without, yet, going into the details of the why, let's talk about the when and the what. I was in an empty hotel gym, fairly late at night, in Dallas, after a couple of days of hellishly stressful work and confrontation, which appeared to be unleashing a new, charged power of mind and affect. I stared at myself wonderingly in the mirror, freshly enthralled at the rapidly clarifying personality that was emerging from the broken shell of depression. I didn't feel as if I was undergoing an actual personality change, so much as I believed that the inner, true Keith - the person I'd have become much earlier had I not arrived at my new school, age seven, as a shrunken shell - was only now tearing off the cloying embryonic matter, and bellowing aloud at my arrival in a new world, a world ripe for my picking.

As I stared at myself in the mirror, I saw my eyes blazing with fire. It felt as if there were a fecund, controlled explosion going on in my mind and body. I'd begun mulling over the idea of writing a novel about a man who recovers from a life-time of depression to become a superstar, and, as I worked out, ideas began to flood my brain. In between sets of bicep curls, I sent myself text messages on my cell phone with whole sentences from the opening chapter of the book I was dreaming up. Rereading it now, it was grandiloquent stuff, but it fully embodied my state of mind then.

> *This is not an ordinary story. For one thing, it's not about me. For another, my subject asked me not to reveal my identity, mainly, I think, because he hasn't told the story to anyone else. So please forget the usual conventions of irony, creative story telling or other fashionable notions of narrative. You will not find out much about me, except in the conclusion, where I may indulge you with a clue or two. About me, that is.*

> *Everything that follows is true, yet shaded to protect the innocent. It's a story that I've put together through numerous meetings with ... what name shall I give him? For now, let's just call him K, as a tribute to one of my own literary heroes, in Kafka's "The Trial".*

> *His is a story about transformation. One thinks of Kafka again: his novella "The Metamorphosis"; yet in this case the protagonist becomes not a huge bug, but something far different...*

That night, I drove to the gay neighbourhood to explore. I'd turned into what I saw as a bewitching master-manipulator of people's affections. I felt I could charm anybody, always knowing the precise words, intonation and body language to win them over.

I played pool with a new buddy, then got back to my hotel around one, and wrote down more ideas for my novel. They were bubbling up almost too fast for me to write down, and I didn't have much to write on. I quickly used up the hotel notepads, the brochure that listed the hotel amenities, and even the dust-cover of one of the books, *Fiasco*, about the Iraq war, I was reading. I couldn't sleep because of the writing. Whole sentences would form in my mind, begging to be written down, not all of them related to the novel, but documenting what I saw as the life-changing transformation underway inside of me.

I've had no fatigue nor depression nor fear of almost any kind in weeks. Is that just feeling high energy, or is it a sign of true change and a fulfillment of my emotional, professional and social potential?

I've been incredibly successful in bringing people to my point of view. Almost the whole team at work is on my side, despite my violent clash with the tech-lead, and I've been told I'm a genius. Is that the case, or do I just talk a lot? I can juggle an almost infinite number of balls at the same time, and not get angry, stressed or hot under the collar unless pushed too far, like I was when I walked off the job the other day to save myself from an aneurysm.

I can charm anybody, and mold their actions. Is that megalomania, or is it just high emotional intelligence? I can sound incredibly boastful and conceited. Or is that just supreme self-confidence, an awareness of my talents, and a desire to be understood? My mind is always running a million miles an hour. Is that organic insanity? Or is it just an abnormally fertile mind?

I'm in a war zone with no intermission. I feel normal limits don't apply to me and that I could quite literally do anything I put my mind to. I can communicate quickly, cogently, and with great facility, exactly to the point. Or do I just like the sound of my own voice?

I can cope with all and every social situation without fear. I can make new friends easily, and can flirt with the self confidence and bravado of a gigolo. Moreover, I can do all of this simultaneously, after little sleep, and along with stress that should be disabling.

Every few minutes while I'm writing these very lines, I'll stop writing and say, 'I should really try to get some sleep.' I'll take another huge swig of wine, conscious that it's 2.30 or so, and that I have to do some work in the morning before checking out of my hotel and flying home. Nonetheless, the very next second, I pick up my pen again, before the spilled wine even dries on my cheeks, and my writing becomes increasingly sleepy and feverish as the Xanax, Ambien and wine hit home.

(I believed I'd taken several Xanax, and was shocked that it wasn't working. I later realized I'd mixed up my Xanax with Ibuprofen, because, you know, the green gel caps just look like those little blue pills.)

Miraculously, I close my eyes. Will I ever shut up? But this is priceless, even if insane. Finally, I brush my teeth, recognizing suddenly that I haven't done so in three days. It's just my bad luck that I'm reading "Parallel Worlds" by Michio Kaku, a truly insane summing up of the most recent cosmological theories. If my own ideas aren't enough to keep my mind spinning, Kaku's imaginative multiverses wind me up.

I'm still writing, fading into oblivion. When, oh when, will the final word of the night arrive?

It's not so late. I can have a good night's sleep. Nothing seems of consequence: brushing my teeth, getting addicted to alcohol, Xanax, Ambien, dying, going to war; nothing, that is, except losing Ben, being dishonorable or vile, or losing my mind. I no longer need validation, least of all an open relationship, as I'd thought last weekend. Nothing makes me tired. I am seemingly Superman, or am I completely off my rocker?

I've been aware all week that I've certainly been talking an awful lot. Everybody I meet – and I mean everybody – looks at me with a mixture of respect, curiosity and ... wariness. But surely if I was insane, everyone would give me a wide berth. Nobody did. Is the fact I'm even having these types of thoughts an indication of genius, or of insanity? In fact, right now, I feel destined for huge things; I feel I can change people's lives permanently. Give back to everybody after forty years of neediness. But will they think I'm crazy, self-serving, arrogant, and egotistical? I have no use for these vices, but as I write I'm clueless as to whether this is insanity talking or something else.

... It's the next morning. Is my brilliance still here? Were the scribbles of last night those of a

Broken Whole

maniac? Reading them now, I find I'm unable to decide. It doesn't matter anymore if it makes sense, because I realize I've red-shifted once more, overnight.

I was like a rolling stone gathering mass; or a speeding train, racing ever faster on a dangerous curve. And we all know what can happen to speeding trains, particularly in slow motion. Yet just months earlier I'd been in the depths of depression, an overly familiar illness which had robbed me of the opportunity to be myself, and had reoccurred with ... well ... depressing frequency ever since my first episode not long after moving to San Francisco at the age of twenty-seven. Within a couple of months of moving there, I met Xavier, a Mexican artist. He came from an upper-middle class family and was worldly, charming, witty, animated, and a bit of a snob (hence his name Xavier, pronounced the French way, rather than Javier). He could be cruel and viciously sarcastic to other people, and I'd have to later privately apologize to friends I'd introduced him to, as if apologizing for our relationship, saying, 'He's not like that when we're alone together.'

Things began well enough – his outgoing, adventurous nature balanced my more reserved, cautious one, and I found myself letting my hair down. But as the honeymoon period passed into the fall, old issues of mine began to surface, and our ability to relate comfortably to one another withered, choked by my jealousy and insecurity. We decided – senselessly – that living together would solve all our problems, and rented a small, inexpensive apartment near the Haight. It was a place I'd grow to hate: not only were his paintings (most of which depressed me with their tortured subject matter and violent colour) all over the walls, but he gradually – perhaps subconsciously to make up for what was missing in our relationship – began to buy plants, which ate up more and more of our precious floor space. Being a big guy, I'd inevitably brush against his precious plants now and again, which provided us fodder for our popular argument: 'Mind the plants!' 'How can I avoid them, they're taking up the whole fucking apartment!'

I would use the words 'I love you,' to him, and, at the time, believed them. Yet, looking back, it's clear to me now that it was more of a lethal mixture of insecurity and sexual obsession stoked by his narcissistic manipulation. As we grew used to each other, he started to use his cruel wit against me occasionally, and became very controlling of every tiniest bit of my behaviour. I have always had this unconscious habit of whistling whatever tune happens to be helplessly lodged in my brain (which is why I hate supermarket shopping, since you're more than likely to be subjected to *Gold* by Spandau Ballet), and I was doing so one day when we were driving to the movies. He asked me to stop, which I did temporarily, only to start up again, without thinking about it, seconds later. Next time, when he asked me to stop whistling, his words were brutal. I stopped the car, got out, and walked home.

Xavier liked to go clubbing a lot more than I did, so I'd let him go by himself even though I knew it would consign me to hours of sleeplessness where I'd be groaning, and quite literally tearing at my hair in agonies of jealousy with thoughts of him dancing shirtless with other men. Staring at his depressing paintings made it that much worse. When he'd come home, I'd pretend to be asleep; it was part of my code never to say anything about it. It was only after we broke up that I found out that my jealous imagination had been couched in reality – he really had been cheating on me, regularly.

I became consumed with either envy or jealousy; I couldn't tell which since they both had the same bitter taste. I was envious that Xavier could be so free with showing his body, and also jealous of the attention that it would inspire. I'd secretly check his gym bag to see what he was wearing at the gym, knowing that even if I verified he was wearing nothing but skimpy shorts (in the early nineties, you could still work out shirtless at his gym), there was no way I'd own up to checking his bag. I was torturing myself.

I was feeling strangely tired all the time, and this, combined with the raging jealousy, spiraled me helplessly into a serious clinical depression, something I'd never experienced before. It seemed as if everything was whirling around me inside a tornado, bits and pieces of my life caught up in the cruel currents; I couldn't grab on to anything substantial to ground me. I broke up with Xavier, and told him I didn't love him. Being involved with a Latin artist is a risky proposition, bringing with it a double load of drama. So I wasn't particularly surprised when he started to stalk me. He threatened to send naked photos of me to my parents (take my advice – never let your partner take naked photos of you), so I tried to have him deported. After that – and a screamingly irate call from his mother - I didn't seem him for a few weeks, and hoped for the best. But I came home from work one night to find him crying on my doorstep, and, like an idiot, I let him in. After coming out of the bathroom, I found him in my bed wearing nothing but a grin. I actually laughed out loud to be living a sitcom in real time. As I attempted to throw him out, his mercurial nature showed itself with hysteric bawling, and, before I pushed him out the door, a threat of suicide. Though Xavier was never deported (and never committed suicide), I did, eventually, free myself both from him and the depression, the latter with the help of Prozac. But, in the words of Tolkien, the whole affair had laid a doom on my life, and, for the next decade, I became something of a hermit, eventually succumbing to chronic fatigue syndrome, to add to the intermittent depressions that returned through my thirties.

In the first draft of this book, you'd have spent several chapters with me wallowing in the mud that made up most of my thirties, reading chapter titles like *Hermit*. In the name of charity, however, I'll just move right to the end of that period, where, I'm happy to report, I'd pulled my life together again, staging a complete recovery from chronic fatigue syndrome, with the help of just about the only doctor in the country who understood it, Jon Kaiser in nearby Mill Valley. I re-entered society with a vengeance, finding myself dating several guys at the same time, and making new friends left, right and centre. My depression was still there in the background, but it no longer controlled my life. I'd been single for ten years, and had dated on and off the old fashioned way – that is through the Internet. But I'd ultimately reached a point where I was comfortable at staying single. (Why does that phrase always sound just a little pathetic?) Many of the barriers that had held my personality in chains for so long had been broken down. My gut and intellect were becoming more aligned with reality, and, on most days, except when depression was around, I liked the person I'd become: a warm, creative, good-natured, bright, charming, charismatic, likeable guy, I thought.

    My mother, who was a fount of useful sayings and words of wisdom, had once said: 'If you're happily working in the garden, sooner or later somebody will look over the garden fence.' (I can't imagine in what context she said this to me, since we at no time in my life ever discussed my romantic life.) But like in so many other things, she was right. In the spring of 2004, I met Ben, a sexy, charming, brilliant, witty doctor doing research into infectious diseases at UCLA. Although I admired his intellect, his staggeringly outgoing nature, and his huge smile, not to forget his tight, lickable biceps, our dating staggered along for a while, largely due to the failure on my part to get my heart into gear.

    Ben was responsible for keeping the light alive, and touched me with a card sent to me after what I'd perceived to be a disastrous date. I'd gone into a short-term depression which really only lasted a matter of weeks, and was probably caused by temporarily discontinuing the hormone supplements which had aided my recovery from chronic fatigue syndrome. We'd spent a weekend together in Palm Springs, and, although I'd completely concealed my depression, it had coloured all of our time together. At a pool party, I gamely carried a laughing Ben on my back, as I waded through the pool, meanwhile feeling utterly dead inside. But Ben wrote 'You're a beautiful person, inside and out,' and ended with a quotation from Yeats:

'I have spread my dreams beneath your feet. Tread softly...'

It brought tears to my eyes, yet the next day I don't believe thoughts of him crossed my mind at all. When love finally announced itself, a couple of months after my minor depression had ended, it was on gay pride weekend in San Francisco. He was just returning from seeing his family in Singapore, and I picked him up at SFO, took him home, and stripped him naked on the padded L-shaped bench which wrapped around the sun-filled windows of my living room. It was unbelievably erotic, and I was suddenly aware of being inundated with a hunger and passion I barely recognized. Ben must have noticed it, although I didn't immediately say anything about it. We did however stop and stare at each other in the sunlight, and I grinned. 'It doesn't get better than this.' That night, I cried during the middle of sex, which rather worried a surprised Ben. (And rather worried a surprised Keith too.) I couldn't really understand the wash of emotion sloshing around inside my brain. Completely unintentionally, during sex, I said 'I love you'. But, gentleman that Ben is, he politely pretended he hadn't heard it, since sex-bed confessions are notoriously unreliable.

That night, we stayed out dancing at a gay pride party until four-thirty, spending the last half hour of that time dancing slowly, wrapped around each other, in our own separate world, having an intimate conversation. As horribly corny as it sounds, if I attempt to recall those moments, I could swear there was nobody else on the dance-floor but us. Ben mentioned, half jokingly, that maybe I wouldn't like him so much if I knew him warts and all. After five years, I have yet to find many warts on him, but, that night, I mentioned that I was covered in warts too, and he asked me to name one. I joked that I really should wear a t-shirt saying "Not tested on boyfriends." Then I took a deep breath, and decided it was time to tell him that I'd suffered from depression for many years. I felt suddenly that perhaps telling him this was not, after all, a sign of weakness, but maybe more of strength: that I'd been able to live with my depression, and hadn't let it become my master.

At the Pride festival, on another perfect, warm day, we lay in the sun for a while, and I reveled not only in the feeling of the sun on my bare torso, but also in the new-found, wholly unexpected reality that I was in love for the first time in at least ten years, and, for the first time, it with somebody who also loved me. That Ben was obviously completely and strongly attracted to me, and had no hesitation about telling me, was having a remarkable effect on me. For the first time in a relationship with an equal, I didn't feel challenged by my own insecurities, and I was finding that I was totally uninhibited sexually. The reality of his love for me was even now just sinking in. I felt walls collapsing all about me as I thought through the implications: the vista of holiday weekends alone with my tuna melts, that I'd thought my lot in life as an adult, was obliterated. I somehow knew from that moment something I'd have previously thought impossible: I would never be alone again.

I wrote in my online photo-journal:

> *It was really only this morning, Monday, after our incredible weekend together, that I realized just how deeply I've fallen for Ben. As I try to concentrate on my work, just thinking about him again sends waves of chemicals coursing through my body. Ben has always been uninhibited and courageous about showing and telling his feelings. Hitherto, I've been afraid that his feelings, which I wasn't sure about returning, could scare me away. Now, in the space of a weekend, I'm beginning to feel the reverse, and think that I might easily come on too strong to him now. Where have all these emotions been hiding all these years?*

Broken Whole

Ben rapidly became, in my mind, the sort of guy everybody wanted to know and go home with at a party. When I was with him, I felt as if it was Christmas every day. But there was hard bed-rock supporting the rush of endorphins. The cement of our relationship was not the sex (although it was the best I'd ever had), it was our shared interests in one another's lives. Ben is a scientist and, although his specialty is virology, he reads widely in other fields I'm interested in. For example, we both consume with great avidity the latest books on cosmology. And I've read at least a few pages from a book almost every single day of my life, since I was in the cradle, ranging from 18th-early 20th century British and American literature, to history, and science. I'm also very interested in the arts, particularly classical music (from Mahler through Stravinsky to Adams, back to Mahler, and more Mahler), modern dance, modern art and film. And I discovered that Ben enjoyed it when I explained the writer's devices in the book I was reading, or when I pointed out to him the structure of a movie. And I did so – I hope – without sounding like Max von Sydow lecturing Barbara Hershey in *Hannah and Her Sisters*. (Movies are always the same, if you watch them with a knowing eye: a hook to grab your attention, followed by a scene introducing our hero in his native element, and then the statement of his goal. Fortune seems to be smiling on our hero, until a plot twist has him losing the girl. A late, mad dash to the airport to head off her imminent departure usually follows, and there ensues the release of having our hero meet his goal, and change for the better, in the process. This also happens to be the plot of this book, except there is no mad dash to the airport. There is a mad dash to the psych ward, however, come to think of it, no pun intended.)

The stars felt aligned for us, wherever we were. We saw each other every weekend, either in LA or San Francisco, and the weather was always sparkling. Even when Ben visited me during a business trip to New York in July, there was no humidity. And we did all the things star-crossed lovers do in movies, such as eating a huge room-service dinner, with ice cream and strawberries for desert, then deserting desert for the sex bed. We did everything except lick ice cream off each other's faces (a rather obscure romantic-comedy motif which seems completely icky to me.)

There was even a departure from Venice at sunset. (That's Venice, Italy – with apologies to Europeans for having to underline that point, but there may be Americans reading this book. Apologies to Americans for that snide remark, but really, how many people watching a *Bourne* movie need to be told that Berlin is in Germany?) I'd never been somebody who believed in rapid U-Haul romance, yet, after that once-in-a-lifetime gay cruise together with two of our best friends, in the Mediterranean, which we'd planned long before we fell in love, I drove down to LA from San Francisco one weekend near Halloween, with half of my wardrobe in the back of my SUV, for an experimental stay with Ben at his house in Sherman Oaks. Three weeks later, after twelve years in the city where I thought I was going to live to my dying days, I was calling up a moving company. It helped that I could do my job as a software developer anywhere, and, in any case, my employer had a small office in Century City, not far from UCLA. There had never been the possibility of Ben moving to San Francisco, since he was on tenure track at UCLA.

Even before I moved down to Los Angeles, when I was drowning in the proverbial sea of love, I nonetheless began to re-experience depression; and, worse: my horrible old insecurities and "issues" began to re-emerge. I had a very sexy photo of Ben on my desk, taken on our third or fourth date, showing him in Charmlee Park near Malibu, walking towards me, in the fullness of youthful vitality, just wearing jeans and a shockingly gorgeous smile. And yet every time I looked at it, I felt anxiety and pain. I eventually had to put it face down on my desk. I realize this is hard to understand, and I'm not sure I can even explain it now myself, since such neuroses are foreign to me now, thankfully. Back then, though, other old companions were re-emerging too, such as jealousy, and fear of abandonment. I'm at a loss to explain the latter since I had a rock solid family. It was probably more a fear of rejection, something that was terribly familiar to me from my early teens at school, where I was a miserable misfit.

Ben told me one day, over the phone, that he was eating more protein, and wanted to get bigger, and I felt a tinge of panic. But this wasn't even the worst of my worries. The biggest trigger for depression was something with which I'd struggled all of my adult life: whenever my boyfriend (whether my first true love, Shaun, or later, Xavier, and now Ben) wore something very sexy in public, then I became very jealous. And I'd been unlucky enough to three boyfriends who particularly liked to dress very sexily. It could tear me up inside. Over time I began to be completely unsure whether it was really jealousy; perhaps it was envy that I felt I couldn't wear something like that. More probably, it was a mixture of both, but either way, it caused me much pain and anxiety, particularly given that I was too ashamed of such feelings to admit them to anybody, let alone my boyfriend.

Ben was very adventurous in how he dressed when we went out clubbing. Again, I couldn't say anything. The only controlling mechanism which I could arrive at, now that I was more confident of my own body, was to try to match Ben in dressing sexily, if not even over-take him, so that I could staunch the envy part of the equation. I shopped mercilessly, tracking down dangerously porn-star pants and tightly tailored shirts to out-sexy my boyfriend. But this did nothing to ameliorate the jealousy.

Things came to a head for me one weekend when Ben visited me in San Francisco, a few months before I moved down to Los Angeles. When I saw him unpacking a particularly sexy pair of scandalously low-cut red pants made out of a clinging, thin red material, which he'd brought for clubbing on Saturday night, the bottom dropped out of my stomach. I spent the rest of the weekend, until we actually did go out, worrying about it. Ben was, of course, totally oblivious to this since I never said anything. To top things off, he never ended up even wearing them.

After Ben had left, I talked it over with my therapist, Erika, and we agreed that I had to own up to the issue. I should open myself to Ben, tell him that I didn't in any way want to control him, but were there things we could do as a couple to help diminish my anguish? Thinking about telling Ben and actually telling him were two different things. The next weekend, I told him there was something I wanted to talk about. We sat down on the bed; but each time I approached the brink of explaining to him the issue, I found I just couldn't say it: I felt so ashamed of my own feelings – as if telling him would make me look weak.

Finally, I managed to get it out, in a tortured, breathless, almost inaudible gasp, my voice unrecognizable. It was such a strange idea to Ben that it took quite a long time before he could even understand what I meant. He wasn't, by nature, short on empathy, but he was unusually lacking in introspection, and therefore found it difficult to understand how something like this could preoccupy me so much. We talked it over at length, and although it became clear later that he still didn't even really get it that night, we agreed that we'd have a "no surprises" approach to what we wore to go clubbing: we'd talk about it ahead of time, so that I wouldn't spend the whole weekend worrying.

Before moving down, I'd made Ben promise that we'd be proactive, and find a couples' counsellor. Ben, coming from Asia where therapy is frowned upon, was dead set against it. He felt that it showed that we had problems, when, in fact, to his mind, our relationship was one of perfect ease. But I came down to LA with a three-page list of "issues" about living together. Some of these were ridiculous. For instance, I imagined Ben coming back from work after I'd been home all day – I often worked at home - and not being affectionate with me as I lay on the sofa. (As opposed to now, when he's lucky to get a kiss from me after he walks in the door.) Or that he'd want to watch television all the time, and even keep the sound on during the commercials (which I hated to an almost obsessive extent.) But Ben is a very adaptable and open to compromise, and most of my issues proved to be paper tigers. I never had to raise them either with Ben or with our new couples' therapist, Paul. As for the clothing issue, I think Ben finally only really understood it in a session with Paul. Ben had never seen me cry; in fact I don't think I'd cried at all since my early twenties, when I'd positively wailed after breaking up with Shaun. As Paul led me back to those teenage years where kids would yell out at me across the street because of my height, my big feet, and my ill-fitting clothes, I surprised myself by starting to sob. That was when Ben began to understand.

The issue didn't really go away completely, right then, but it was suddenly manageable. Ironically, I became rather infamous amongst our friends for the way I dressed to go clubbing. I was inspired by Ben's own adventurous nature, a sense of wanting to compete, and a growing sense of how my own rapidly improving physique (driven by unstated competition with Ben) gave me more choices. There was almost a reversal in my understanding of what I could get away with. I used to think that because I was so tall, I couldn't dress in a way that attracted attention. Now I realized that it was exactly because I was so tall that I could get away with clothes that might look outrageous on others. Or at least I'm hoping that's the reason nobody ever told me I looked ridiculous.

I couldn't have plotted an unhappier story about a man's arrival in Los Angeles than what actually happened. Ben's house in the Valley was cold, and dark, and you could always hear the noise from the 101 Freeway almost right behind the back yard. It was the second rainiest winter in Los Angeles history. I'd had an unrealistic expectation of Ben's availability during the months of our long-distance relationship, where we'd spent almost every weekend together, Friday night to Monday morning. But now it was grant-writing season, and Ben had scientific papers which had been on the back-burner while we got to know each other, and were now falling to dust from lack of attention. He'd rarely come home before eight o'clock.

I work for a large software company, usually on big development and integration projects. But I can often go long period – months – without any project work. To most people, this sounds like a happy situation; after all, I still get paid. You mean you get paid to do nothing, my friends ask incredulously? In San Francisco I'd often used these times to develop my outside interests, such as film-making, and website-development. I had a very popular gay website, which included an extensive online photo-journal, and maintaining both the site and my correspondence with fans had taken up much of my time. But about six months after I'd fallen in love with Ben, I realized that the website, and the attention I received from fans, had been filling a hole in my life that had now been completely closed over. As a result, though, I no longer had the website to fall back on as a constant source of creative work to keep my mind occupied when not busy with work.

Around the time I met Ben, I'd been living, all expenses paid, in Manhattan for six months, on the most complex, demanding and fulfilling project of my career. Ten months later, when I moved to live with Ben, the project was cancelled, and I was suddenly at a loose end. This went on throughout the winter. I didn't know what to do with myself. I had an office in Century City in an executive suite, where there was nobody from my company and hence no colleagues. I'd sit and stare out of the floor-to-ceiling window for hours, in a deadened slump, or plough maniacally, for hours, through new web sites like *Hot-or-Not,* and *MySpace*, downloading photos of hot guys. Even now, whenever I drive past Century City on the way to UCLA, I feel a shudder of remembered unhappiness – the whole area is coloured (if such a word is even appropriate) by depression. Many days I'd not go into the office, and would stay home. I worked out twice a day, and ran four times a week, putting more effort into improving

Broken Whole

my body than bettering my mood. Most household chores would fall my way, since I had so much free time. Some days I'd drive ten featureless blocks in the eternally flat lands of the Valley to Target, then ten in another to go to Home Depot. I felt like a Valley housewife. Maybe next, I'd take to readying Ben's slippers in anticipation of his coming home, and mixing him a martini.

Unrelieved depression has a corrosive effect on your cognition. For instance, I knew few people in LA, and, in any case, those few friends all worked during the day. As a result of spending way too much time in almost complete isolation, I could feel so easily abandoned. I'd spend a long day just waiting for the time Ben would call; then I knew we'd be together soon – that the loneliness would end. On those nights when Ben called to say he had to work late, and could I go to the gym without him, I felt almost overwhelmed with hurt. I felt ashamed of my emotional dependence on him, which only served to intensify the depression. It was a curse that would steal the life from our relationship, I believed, but I was helpless to counteract it in any meaningful way.

On my worst days, everything bothered me. Ben's thoughts were frequently tuned to his scientific work when we were driving together. I'd say something to him, and it would be as if he didn't hear it. Even though I understood that he was so involved in his own internal thought processes that he genuinely didn't consciously hear me, I took it personally, each time. At the gym, Ben would look at himself in the mirror, and sometimes even dance along to the music for a second or two. I'd want to tell him to stop, because his spontaneity and gaiety made me feel badly about myself. I'd feel a vast emptiness sweep over me the moment the door closed behind Ben on his way out to work. I even felt pain when he fell asleep at night – that I was to be absent in his presence until morning. I'd be competitive and insecure about the smallest things, not just my body. If we drove separate cars, met up at the gym, then drove home, I'd cut corners just to beat him to our house. Ben used moisturizer on his body, and I felt bitter that I couldn't do likewise without breaking out in acne. I don't tell these things with any pride – in fact, it's painful to reveal them (although much less so now that I've left these neuroses behind me). My saving grace back then (for it truly would have been death to our relationship) was that I never acted on my feelings to try to control Ben. The downside of this approach was that it kept everything bottled up.

Depression is an insidious worm which can eat away, sight unseen, at the base of a relationship. Because you typically have no feelings at all, when depressed, the expression of feelings from others is almost painful to bear. You know that you can't return them, so you're faced with feigning it, repelling it, or bearing it without affect, hoping that the other person won't notice the coldness of your response. In a close relationship with somebody like Ben, who by nature expresses feelings easily, spontaneously, and naturally, then the depression itself can arouse expressions of care and sympathy, thus compounding the feedback loop. So you don't talk about it. You rarely express, even to the person you share a life with, how wretched you feel, during the worst times. You know that your partner's empathy comes from nowhere but a good and generous place in their heart, but it nevertheless leaves you feeling even more barren than had nothing been expressed in the first place, since you're left feeling "damaged". And you yourself, of course, are held back from initiating any expression of love or affection. I always worried that this dynamic would leach the colour from our relationship, but couldn't see what I could do to change things. Fortunately, I can say that my partner is extremely long suffering, although you've probably drawn that conclusion on your own by now.

It might sound, from all this, as if it would have been impossible for us to have an enjoyable relationship. In the worst parts of the depression, there was no doubt that it was tough for Ben, since on the one hand he felt helpless to offer assistance, while on the other hand, he felt bad for himself that he wasn't helping me. He almost felt as if he were to blame. But there were long periods where depression receded to the point where those little things didn't bother me as much, and there was enough solidity to our relationship in other ways that it wasn't immediately threatened by the secret neuroses that frequently governed my mood.

One of the conditions of my giving up my life and circle of friends in San Francisco was that Ben would sell his house, and we'd buy one together. The Valley, where Ben was living when I met him, was verboten, since I've long had an abhorrence of the suburbia embodied by the San Gabriel Valley. And twelve years living in the Castro in San Francisco had made me even less prepared to come across housewives in sweatpants at the supermarket. Just before going to London at Christmas, where my family met Ben for the first time, we moved out of Sherman Oaks into – temporarily – a large apartment across the freeway from Universal Studios. The rain had raised the water table, and we came home from London to find the kitchen, bedroom and bathroom under several inches of water. (It was immediately after the tsunami in South-East Asia, and it didn't escape our ironic eye that the sand-bags we bought had 'Made in Indonesia' stamped on them.) Not only did our bedroom smell of skunk, but our two big dogs, Indira, and Brewster, had got into several boxes of chocolate truffles we'd received for Christmas, and subsequently thrown up brown bile all over the carpet in the living-room. (Chocolate does not agree with dogs. Especially when eaten in large quantities.) I began to have dark thoughts that I should have stayed in San Francisco. One day Ben came home to find me staring out of the window. I turned around, and he asked me what was wrong. 'I'm lonely.' It just slipped out, along with a sob. 'I've left my entire support network back in San Fran.' I looked around the living room, still with brown stains on the floor, and into the bedroom floored with sand bags and planks under a couple of inches of rain. I almost said 'Is this what I moved down for?'

Soon after, we bought a beautiful, sunny house in the eastern hills of Hollywood, just on the edge of the valley, looking into a ravine which sloped up to the hill on which sat the Hollywood sign. I was terrified when the LA Times was delivered the first morning: it was the Valley edition. But a quick check of the map confirmed we were in Hollywood. I'd later wonder what I was thinking when we bought the house, since it meant that for the first time since childhood I'd be living somewhere with no street life, where you couldn't walk to a café. Even in the daytime, there's almost complete silence. In any event, not even the adventure of building a new home served to pull me out of what was now my worst depression since my first, in my late twenties.

I finally got a new project at work, and my depression ameliorated a little. The work was of little social utility, since it involved developing a software system for targeted bulk-mailing campaigns. My smart and sexy boyfriend professor, on the other hand, was saving the world. He was doing this incredibly nifty experiment in which mice got implanted with human tissue in their kidney regions. This somehow grafted with their kidneys, and soon, human blood cells were coursing through their bloodstreams. Next, they took a sample of the matter from the transformed kidney, and injected it into the tail veins of the poor mice, and, eventually, this found its way to their bone marrow. This had the effect of spurring a wholesale chimerical regeneration of various parts of their bodies, so that they were left with, amongst other things, a human immune system, and a half-formed human hand jutting out of their backs. Professor *Frankenstein* boyfriend - hadn't invented this technique, but he was the first person to validate the original procedure. More important, it allowed him to infect the long-suffering mice with viruses that would otherwise only infect humans, and test his potentially wonder compound, the one which might make his career, on them. (I was joking, by the way, about the human hand coming out of their backs.)

Broken Whole

By this time, we were temporarily down to one car since we'd crashed his sporty Volvo convertible. (Ben was asleep so it wasn't his fault. I was asleep too. Unfortunately, I was also driving). I also wrecked three parked cars, and, incredibly, we both walked away with nothing more than slightly wrenched necks. Having just one car, I'd have to drive him if I wanted to avoid being stuck at home all day with no escape transportation (since it was so infradig to take local buses, which I'd had to do all throughout my childhood.) On the drive, I'd often be completely silent, answering Ben's comments and questions with monosyllables. So Ben would talk about his work, telling me about his grant proposals and ideas. We both recognized that we were unusually lucky in each having a boyfriend who was an intellectual equal. I could get the drift of most of what Ben explained. But if I tried to share his excitement, as far as my sodden grey matter would allow, I couldn't hide from the part of me that felt shamefully embittered. When I'd been tech-lead on a major work project in New York, when I first got to know Ben, I'd done the best work of my career, and had become regarded by my peers as a strong leader and problem-solver. I was taking this newly reaffirmed self-knowledge into my new project. Although it had unappealing ends, the means were interesting, posing many complex logical and technical problems. And it was for one of the foremost financial institutions in the world. In response to Ben's excitement about his work, I'd try to explain to him the challenges of what we were doing. He'd listen patiently, and ask questions to show his interest. I was fully aware that he knew that I had nothing to prove to him, and that he greatly respected my intelligence; but there was a chip on my shoulder about having an occupation that didn't match what I saw as my intellectual potential. I'd quit two PhD programs in my early twenties, for personal reasons, despite my early intention to be a scientist, and I knew that if I'd stayed in academia, I could have been doing the sort of important work Ben was doing. Instead, I visualized myself in my fifties, still a software-developer, albeit a highly successful and well-paid one, now being the oldest person in the room at meetings I recoiled at the vision. I still felt that great things could come to me, but I couldn't see the path.

In a lull in my project, I got a small part playing an alien extra in a big science-fiction movie[1], and Ben was unusually excited for me. When you're in depression, it effortlessly knocks down your defenses, and you become vulnerable, and prickly. So when Ben told me how happy he was for me, a tiny little voice inside me made me compare my big exciting thing with his own work saving the world one mouse at a time, and I felt, suddenly, a little pathetic. I couldn't help saying to myself softly inside my head 'Of mice and men, indeed' Darkly, I even suspected Ben of overstating his excitement in order to make me feel better.

As with all things, my depression came to an end, like storm clouds rapidly fleeing a blue sky in the ever changing weather of my home British Isles. My hide regained its thickness and all the darts of pain borne out of "my issues" became so much less piercing. But I was still suffering from my other long-term illness, Sehnsucht, a wonderful German word with no equivalent in other languages, which means an ineffable longing for you know not what. I was forty, and I still didn't know what I wanted to be when I grew up.

Eighteen months later, newly recovered from another depression with the aid of the antidepressant Lexapro, I was

---

[1] It was the *Star Trek* reboot, requiring a seventeen-hour shoot, mostly overnight, at the Port of Long Beach. My scene was completely cut. Otherwise I'd point you to the six-foot-six alien with a green, globular head. Oh, there was another member of my species who turned out also to be six-foot-six, but I was the pretty one, since he had a wicked slash across his cheek. I did this little bit of business with a rock, which I thought very clever. I hoped that wasn't why the scene was cut. The deleted scene did resurface in the DVD, but try as I might, I cannot see myself in the background, carrying my rock. To my chagrin, however, my next-door neighbor appears very prominently in one of the other deleted scenes.

Broken Whole

in that Dallas gym, relishing the full-blown mania which I'd interpreted as a mind-blowing reawakening. After having been through so much darkness, you can imagine the immense joy with which I greeted my new-found powers to be anybody, and to do anything I wanted. I'd felt, all my life, on account of being so tall, and my relentlessly introspective nature, to be *other than*. I'd never belonged anywhere. But now all that was changed. I finally knew I was going to be *in*. And, not surprisingly, the siren call of achievement that so disturbed me during depressions now seemed like a wondrous thing.

In the days and weeks ahead – the period occupying most of the rest of this book - I was to pursue many dreams. I began the planning for building a gay super-club in West Hollywood from the ground up. I booked a corner suite at the W in San Francisco for four weeks, and intended to hire the best ghost writer available to help me finish my book. Worst of all, just a few days after getting home from Dallas, on the morning of the nightmarish day whose aftermath is portrayed in the prelude to this book, I walked out of my house believing I'd uncovered something that could both cause major changes in the world economy, and make me and all my friends and family rich beyond comparison. I sincerely believed I was the most intelligent person who'd ever lived.

You might ask yourself, is he making all this up? Is he crazy? How could anybody think such things of themselves? And what was this idea that could change the world? Those things will be described in this book, but I can't promise they'll be any more understandable – or believable, unless you can see it through the prism of mania, either self-experienced or by witnessing it in an intimate.

I'm *not* "crazy"; at least, neither right now, nor at any time since 2006. However, I suppose that it depends upon how you define the word "crazy". I *am* crazy, if you consider all serious mental illnesses which have a "bizarre behavior" component to deserve that epithet. But my bipolar disorder has been under full control, as of this writing, for well over three years, thanks to the wonder drugs Depakote and Lamictal. Back then, however, in the late summer of 2006, my mind was kindling into a titanic manic episode that would consume the summer. Coming from acute depression into a world of colour where everything seemed possible by the shear magnetic force of my new self-belief, how was I to know, whilst doing my bar-bell curls in that hotel gym in Dallas, that what felt so amazingly incredibly wonderful was actually the first, untreated, undiagnosed burgeoning of bipolar disorder? I was indeed going crazy.

Which brings me back to who is the real me? Is it the intermittently depressed, but generally level-headed, urbane and well-connected person I'd become after my first horrible winter in Los Angeles? Or is it this shining being in Dallas, who felt fully whole for the first time in his life? Or what about the person writing this book, well recovered from mania, and long free of those piddling insecurities? Or is it none of those? Or all of them? Is the real me's personality gauge set by Lamictal, the mood stabilization drug that keeps me balanced? The mania of 2006 would teach me the harshest lesson of my life – that whether the way I was when manic was the real me or not, I could never let myself be that person without risking my health, my sanity, my relationships, my livelihood and even my life. And that was a pill bitterer by far than Lamictal or Depakote.

Book II – Creativity Run Amok
The Train is Leaving the Station, Dallas, Early August

There were early signals that something strange was creeping about my cranium. In July, we went to England for two weeks, and I demonstrated a new proclivity to explode into a huge temper, reducing Ben frequently to tears. And my wallet was as unleashed as my temper. Ben and I are, by nature (or design), bad with money, and – at least before and through the manic spending binge in the immediate future – have routinely overspent our incomes. But that's not an adequate explanation of why we bought, whilst in another continent, fifty lbs of medieval Scottish armour. I don't remember Ben putting the brakes on, but it was undoubtedly an act announcing a marked departure from reality. And the thing is, I did actually intend to wear it: we had it shipped home to form part of a Halloween outfit. While I was trying on the back-plate and helmet in the quaint tourist store lined with tartan as far as the eye could see, I'm sure the owners must have been thinking to themselves: 'Do they realize it's just for show, and not meant to be worn? Crazy Americans!' (Guilty as charged.) On Halloween night, several months later, I paraded down Santa Monica Boulevard, helmet, red plume, armour, a leather loin cloth, and all..

Back home from the trip, there were two weeks of New York Times to get through, and I insisted on reading every last section. This was another clue about a change in mindset. Manic people can become almost religiously focused. Strangely enough, they can also be flighty and easily distracted, but, once distracted, the laser-like focus just trains on the new object of obsession. Such as my intense desire to purchase *Space Dock*, the actual filmed model of the mushroom-shaped space station built for *Star Trek III: the Search for Spock*. It was being auctioned in a huge sale of

Star Trek props and memorabilia at Christies that summer.[2] The glossy catalogues, which I ordered, listed the expected price as around a thousand dollars, which I thought quite reasonable considering how large *Star Trek* loomed in my psyche. However, that was not the only place it loomed: Space Dock was rather large at 53 by 42 inches, so it was not clear where I planned to put it. (Although it did come with a stand, not to mention a power supply for all the little lights. Perhaps even the space-doors opened at the touch of a button?) It ultimately sold for a little more than the estimate - $78,000. Come to think of, that is almost exactly the amount of money I'd burn through in just a few weeks of mania beginning in August, so I might as well have just bought the darned thing and called it a day.

In late July, after a week of the most intense stress and back-breaking work I'd ever had at work, I flew, exhausted, with Ben to San Diego gay pride to meet friends from San Francisco.

'I'm going to be a superstar,' I told Ben on Saturday night, at a dance club event. In fact, I'd told him several times already. For a couple of years, now, in therapy, I'd had the feeling that if all of the threads in my life could somehow bond together, I'd have a sturdy rope up which to climb. I didn't know where this synergy would come from, whether it would come at all, nor where the rope would lead to. But now I was regularly feeling an unstoppable, surging excitement, and I began to wonder if that moment had arrived. I'd already conquered a problem that had always seemed as insuperable (to me) as the Palestinian conflict, if you'll excuse the comparison. Ever since my childhood I'd been acutely conscious of my body as a separate, skinny entity, flopping by

---

[2] As you might have gathered by now, I'm something of a closet Trekkie. This book marks my official coming out. I assert that I've never worn a *Star Trek* uniform, nor attended a fan conference. However, as a kid, I used to go to sleep desperately hoping that I'd wake up as Mr. Spock.

my side, dragged reluctantly along by an overactive, introspective mind. My mother had always promised that one day 'I'd fill out,' but I didn't expect I'd have to wait until my late thirties. But even after I'd built a gay gym body, there were always moments of self-doubt when I'd unexpectedly see myself in an unfriendly mirror, the bones of the awkward teenager sticking out. But, largely unnoticed, Ben's frequent and obviously heartfelt declarations that he found me sexy, had sunk home. At the party in San Diego, not only did I receive a lot of attention at clubs, I also learned that the attention strangely no longer mattered to me. I'd apparently moved into my body, and now mind and body worked as one, both confident in each other. Even if, as happened, a handsome guy would pointedly and self-consciously ignore me, I'd whisper 'It's just shame' to Ben, who'd laugh at the reference to one of the lessons I'd learned in therapy.

'Most people are ashamed, deep inside ' David, the brilliant cognitive therapist I'd been fortunate enough to find shortly after moving to Los Angeles, had said to me. He'd gone on to compliment me in terms too glowing to repeat here, ending with: 'So I'm going to challenge you. Next time you're walking along the street, and you pass a cute guy: make eye-contact. I'll guarantee that nine times out of ten they'll avert their eyes, and it's shame speaking, every time. But that one time in ten, they'll probably smile.'

I had been tempted to ask David: 'What if the ninety percent are averting their eyes because they think I'm an old troll?' But I held back. The reality was that the decades of doubt about my physicality had dissipated in a matter of weeks, without so much as a whimper.

Mind and body coming together – it was that synergy I'd hoped for, but it had come not in some kind of intellectual fusion, but instead, in a most unexpected form, that of the body. When I told Ben, that weekend in San Diego, that I was on the verge of superstardom, without quite defining what that meant, I was thinking inside that I was on the edge of great things on account of making peace with my body. Yet, I don't suppose I even knew myself what that could entail.

Once the weekend was over, I returned, with a rude shock, to the real world, and, feeling dangerously like a combination of Captain Kirk and Brad Pitt, flew directly from San Diego to Dallas to work, for a week, with my colleagues. I'd always been a good problem solver at work, and now, working sixteen hour days, heading down the slippery slope towards mania, I was intent on solving some intractable problems, both technical and interpersonal. Unfortunately, I'm not at liberty to discuss anything work-related from that week, since I've been told to do so would put me in legal jeopardy, and while I'm not immune to the attractions of selling more books by virtue of a legal scandal, I'd really rather keep my job if it's all right with you. What I can say, though, is that I believed I was discovering in myself qualities of leadership and self-assertion that had either hitherto been dormant due to insufficient self-confidence, or, more likely, were now being stoked by the fire that was beginning to light up inside my brain. And during the first part of the week, this new self-belief was further enabled after talking to David on the phone. I'd called him because I was beginning to feel the burden of work stress and confrontation become unmanageable, and wondered if I should stop putting myself on the line when I felt I had to step in to help steer the project. David told me that he thought I was a born leader. This was exactly the wrong thing for a therapist to say to somebody in the budding phase of mania, although I don't, for one moment, blame David for failing to identify what was going on in my brain during these early stages, since he, like me, was only too glad that I was feeling consistently good after all those years.

The first morning in Dallas, I turned up at work wearing a short-sleeved, barely "business casual", G-Star shirt tailored tightly to my torso and biceps. I'd never been good in the spotlight. In fact, my head tended to shake if I had to speak in public, even if it was just to introduce myself in a small group of strangers, a relic of a traumatic childhood incident where my music teacher had harangued me for thirty minutes in front of a room full of my peers because I'd given up trombone lessons. But now I walked, unperturbed, into my first meeting, to face an accounting for an incendiary action I'd taken on the Friday before heading to San Diego. While I was being grilled, I felt almost preternaturally calm, and was completely certain that I was in the right. Increasingly, I recognized that I was undergoing a remarkable transformation. Nonetheless, I did not feel like I wasn't being myself. Everything seemed to make total sense in my mind. In fact I'd never felt so much at home with myself at any other time in my life.

I was having a particularly difficult clash with one person, and things came to the boil mid-week when the two of us went at each other so violently that I lost my head, and walked off the project. It was a sense of genuine peril that was forcing me to leave. The self-driven belief that there was no level of technical complexity beyond my reach to understand and resolve, and no amount of stress I couldn't handle, had finally thrust up against an immovable object, in the form of the man with whom I was now explosively butting head. In the crisis of the moment, I felt that I literally had to choose between having a heart-attack and smashing his face in. As I packed up my laptop, everybody in the room looked at me wordlessly, open-mouthed, their mouths working like goldfish, unable to believe what they were seeing. It was unheard of for somebody to walk off the job like this. I felt very strange as I left the building and walked to my car in the blazing Dallas sun, not really knowing what I'd done. As I drove back to my hotel, I was beginning to think that the only alternative to going crazy from the stress was to resign.

Your life can hang on a moment's decision. I might well have resigned right there and then, so sure was I, already, due to the ambition and self-believe that comes with manic fervour, that money was not going to be a problem in the future. Now that my judgment of my own abilities is more rational, I know how lucky I am that I chose the only other option available to me that hot day in Dallas: to go crazy. I might have thought this in almost a fanciful way, but I genuinely felt that the stress was near to unmanning me. And I was, actually, in a technical sense, going crazy, since I was spiralling into a manic fit borne of self-imposed stress helped along by a recently begun course of medication (Lexapro). That night I began to consider ideas for a book, and that was why I ended up, late that evening, as I described in the previous chapter, curling biceps in the hotel gym while furiously texting myself whole paragraphs of my book.

Throughout my time in Dallas it seemed that everything conspired to add to my stress level, even the GPS system in my rental-car. I had the misfortune that the major artery along which I needed to drive daily was under construction, and, since I'm directionally challenged, I kept getting horribly lost. The GPS would take thirty seconds to find its new location every time I left the expected route, by which time I'd have taken another wrong turn, and the whole process would begin again while I not-so-silently sat, fuming in rage at the machine, estimating whether the satisfaction of pitching the thing out of the car would be worth the penalty I'd have to pay Avis at the end of the trip.

Another infuriating, recurring feature of that week in Dallas was that people seemed to find me very difficult to understand. I'd ask for, say, a pack of gum, and they'd look at me with mystified eyes as if I was speaking Klingon. I'd read a very unlikely story, while we were in England, about a housewife who'd woken up one morning with a strong Jamaican accent. It was called "Foreign Accent Syndrome". (It's a handy little piece of knowledge to use in refuting Pentecostals when they throw 'speaking in tongues' at you as evidence of the supernatural.) It seemed to be happening to me, now – that is, Foreign Accent Syndrome, not speaking in tongues. In my case, though, my native Geordie accent (the accent of those born on the banks of the River Tyne), freshly recharged, as usual, by having spent a few days with my family in England, refused to depart now, weeks later. Nobody in Dallas could understand the harsh vowels coming from my mouth. To make matters worse, I now knew that both Ben and David were worried that I was becoming manic, which meant that I was especially watching out for people thinking I was nuts. The mute stares of incomprehension I was receiving just fuelled my fear of being thought crazy.

Then there was the toilet-paper problem. In the office in Dallas, the toilet paper had insufficient tensile strength for the holder. When the roll was new, you tried to pull some toilet paper and all you got was half a sheet. The floor was littered with other people's foiled efforts to pull enough paper to wipe their bums. Twenty plus years as a software-developer had trained my mind to spot process problems, and recognize simple solutions. Surely, I thought, this must be a petty inconvenience to everybody, why don't I just tell the building manager that they're using the wrong toilet paper for that particular holder, or that they ought to contact the manufacturer of the toilet-paper holder and tell them their design was flawed. Of course I never followed through on this, because I knew I'd get that incredulous stare of incomprehension. Not everybody sees the world as I do. But this was a symptom of one of my better traits – a yen for process-improvement – revving into a more general, angry feeling that the world was out to get me. Every little bit of technology I used that week seemed to break, or be useless. I swear that even the elevators would seize up whenever I got inside them.

In retrospect, I now know that the manic brain makes strange cognitive errors. For instance, I could be filling in a web-form, and get all bent out of shape because there was no submit button. I might even call someone up on the phone and yell at them. Then either I'd sheepishly notice myself, belatedly, or have somebody else point out to me, the big green button in the corner of the screen saying 'Continue'.

This exemplified itself on the evening of the day I walked off the job when I tried to go to the beautiful gym at one end of the gay village. I had to call the manager several times in order to just get to the lobby of the gym. In my first call, he hadn't told me that it was impossible to see the gym from the street since it was high-up in an office block. When I arrived at the building, it wasn't at all clear which underground parking lot to enter (or it might have been clear, and my brain was too fogged up to figure it out). I got even madder when, after once again calling the gym manager, I determined the right parking lot. I entered this enormous, featureless underground lair, the size of six Trafalgar Squares (hey, somebody has to be the first to break with the football-field cliché), with various exit-doors scattered in the distance, but no signs indicating where I should park in this vastness, let alone how to get into the right building to go to the gym. I looked at my phone – no signal. I had to drive back out of the parking lot to call the manager yet again, barely resisting the urge, at this point, to call him a cretin. That would come later. I felt this raging surge in my head, a sensation I couldn't quite describe – as though the electric current darting about between synapses was suddenly magnified a thousand times.

When I made it up to the lobby, the only sign pointing the way to the gym was next to an elevator. And it was behind locked glass doors. I shook with rage as I called the manager up again. He explained, in his delicate, mincing, southern accent, that he'd have to come down and let me in. When the elevator opened, I saw a squat, dainty-looking African-American man with a look of general self-satisfaction on his face. I offered him – very charmingly I thought, considering his utter inability to be helpful – a suggestion on how to make directions easier for first-time visitors. But the horrible little creature became defensive. Soon, by the time we'd made it into the actual gym, it had grown into a shouting match, and I found myself bellowing after him, as I left, 'Go fuck yourself you pathetic cunt,' while other gym members watched unbelievingly.

I did recognize that my temper was becoming dangerously hair-triggered, but I still believed that it was because of work stress. I also believed that I'd been in the right at the gym. I didn't know it at the time, but this intense focus on seeing my rights validated was going to be the single character trait that would get me into the most serious trouble in the coming weeks.

But I'm getting ahead of myself. After the blow-up at the gay gym, and after another epic story of trying and failing to find both a Gold's Gym that was still open, and a place to buy a bottle of wine to help me calm down now, and aid me in getting to sleep later, I finally ended up working out in the hotel gym. (I could fill a whole chapter just expanding upon that last sentence alone, so convoluted had every seemingly simple act become. But I'm sure you don't want to know about my getting lost in the tiny courtyard between three affiliated hotels, or the misunderstanding with the front-desk of one of the other hotels who confirmed I could get a bottle of wine but waited until it arrived to ask me which room I was in, and no, I couldn't take it if I wasn't actually staying in that hotel.)

The night where I walked off the job, I didn't tell Ben anything, since I knew he was worried about me, and I didn't want to scare him. Although I'd taken what felt like the only rational way out of the most stressful situation of my life, I knew he'd probably see it as another sign that I was becoming manic. I was in the tough position of being simultaneously in dire need of his support and counsel while, on the other hand, too worried about his own anxieties to share with him what had happened. I was trying to shield Ben, whose fears were stoked by his previous manic boyfriend, at a cost to my sanity.

When I returned to the office, the next morning, it turned out that I wasn't unemployed. But I still had to work with the man with whom I'd almost come to blows, and I think I was remarkably civil to him on this, for once, relatively uneventful day, given what had happened the day before. It was, at least, a day relatively free of conflict. And even the elevators seemed more amenable. Yet I was in the eye of the storm.

After a week where I thought I'd already endured the worst crisis of my career, and coped with stress that had almost broken me, Friday was even worse. I worked from my hotel, and was supposed to check out at noon to go to the airport. Really, how bad could things get alone in a hotel bedroom?

I got up at nine, and waded once more into the thick of things. I hadn't showered since Tuesday. I don't think I'd even brushed my teeth since Wednesday morning – I'd been so short of time due to the relentless work, and the sudden driven need I had to express myself in writing, that I'd had to make choices between sleep and hygiene. Or between having a heart attack or a nervous break-down. Or resign of course. My room was a complete mess – work, gym and play clothes left where I'd dropped them each night before crawling into bed. And I had a noon checkout; yet I couldn't seem to gain control over the flurry of emails, and cell-phone calls. Noon came, and I'd already called for a late check-out but still couldn't get off my laptop. I was buried too deep to see that I was doing this to myself.

Then it was one o'clock, and the final confrontation came in the form of an insane request, by email, from my nemesis. Even now, long past the time at which I should have just started saying no, I still didn't give up on rational persuasion. I was still capable, I felt, of juggling all the balls hurled at me. I emailed him to let him know that I'd long since run out of time to check out of my hotel, and that I was far from being the only person who could fulfill his request, and then I prepared to log off. I should have. But before I could do so, another email popped into my inbox, and, helplessly, I clicked it open. It was another unrelenting request from the person I was now beginning to think was deliberately trying to goad me into a rash action.

I'd already made threats about resigning, but I tried one last email to try to get this man to see common sense, albeit in a trenchant email that spelled out clearly what I truly thought of him. I'd made what I thought was an endless effort to appease him, but I now believed he might no longer be in his right mind. This time, after sending the email, despite the lateness of the hour, I stood at my desk, car keys in my hand, everything packed except my laptop, waiting for his response. I didn't even have to open his email because the response was in the subject line, and was a blunt refusal to accommodate me.

I was shaking with rage and stress. I didn't know what to do. In retrospect, of course, I can see that I'd brought a lot of this on myself. My growing mania was magnifying already strong beliefs that I felt I could solve every problem, and manage a large number of complicated tasks at the same time. I was being driven crazy, trying to do the impossible, much like an archetypical computer in the original Star Trek, pushed to self-implode by relentless logic chopping from Captain Kirk. There might even have been smoke coming out of my ears.

I'd already placed one emergency call to David, as well as to my psychiatrist. Finally, in a panic, unable to call Ben for fear of worrying him, I called my best friend, Dean, a tall, smart, handsome, lovely man of about my age, back in Los Angeles. He spoke in tones of measured calm.

'Keith, I was once in a situation like this. I was lucky enough to talk to a friend. He told me to just switch everything off, and walk away.'

I confess I was almost crying at this point. But I thought it through, grasping at the potential of escaping what seemed like an impossible position so easily.

'You can't win right now,' Dean said, 'And if you go any further you're going to do something you'll regret.'

I let my breath out.

Dean probably saved my career. He was able to see what was blindingly obvious: that nobody should put up with this, and I didn't have to. I followed his advice, not responding to the email, and briefly emailed a colleague asking him to take care of the trivial matter that had brought things to such a head. I sent out a group email saying that I was logging off, and then shut off my laptop and cell-phone. It was all so suddenly clear that I could have done this hours earlier, and hurt myself and my career prospects so much less.

Because my flight was now delayed until late afternoon, I had time to go back to the gay village again and relax. It was one hundred degrees, but the tension had all drained out of me, and not even the heat bothered me. I got a gift for Ben, and bought myself a beautiful leather-bound writing book, and started writing in it over a late, white tablecloth lunch at The Melrose, a gorgeous, boutique hotel at the end of the gay village.

Once I arrived at the airport, there was more "mind-confusion" whereby I ended up taking the wrong bus from the car-rental station, and had to return in a mad-dash to take a different bus. Although I missed my flight, the people at the Admirals Club were all smiles and helpful assistance, and I took their rapport with me as confirmation of what I saw as my markedly increased facility with people (excluding my obstinate work colleague, obviously). I was accommodated in first-class on the next flight out. Moreover, the club even had a spa-like private bathroom with a shower, where I could change out of the clothes I'd been sweating in during all of my rushing around. The ordeal was finally over.

I spent my remaining time in the Admirals Club trying to decide what to tell Ben. Because it would be possible to portray things as if I'd once again walked off the job, I really didn't know whether I would have a position or not on Monday. I decided, finally, come what may, I'd just pretend to work at home next week until the dust cleared, and Ben wouldn't need to know anything.

The borderline between a hyper-charged, magnetic, accomplished individual and an out-of control clinical maniac seems broad. That week I'd become aware of strengths and abilities I'd never known I'd had. But on which side of the borderline was I? I'd always been high-functioning, impatient, multitasking, and good at solving problems, yet it seemed that it was these qualities, electrically intensified, that had brought me to this juncture. Although I felt that my behaviour, up until the breaking point on Friday, had just been the final, long delayed inheritance of my birthright, made possible by the terminal dissipation of depression, I had in fact entered the surging river of mania. I'd stood up – as I have always done, but this time at great cost to myself – for what I'd believed was right, but I'd apparently disengaged the governing mechanism that kept a balance between the search for justice and common-sense.

On the flight home, I wrote on the first page of the leather book I'd bought in the gay village: 'The Day', thinking that for years to come I'd know what that day was: the worst, the most intense day of my life. Right.

It's Karma, the week after Dallas.

> *Manic Episode*
> *DSM IV Criteria*

A) *A distinct period of abnormally and persistently elevated, expansive or irritable mood, lasting at least 1 week (or any duration if hospitalisation is necessary)*

B) *During the period of mood disturbance, three (or more) of the following symptoms have persisted (four if the mood is only irritable) and have been present to a significant degree:*

   1. *inflated self-esteem or grandiosity*
   2. *decreased need for sleep (e.g., feels rested after only 3 hours of sleep)*
   3. *more talkative than usual, or pressure to keep talking*
   4. *flight of ideas or subjective experience that thoughts are racing*
   5. *distractibility (i.e., attention too easily drawn to unimportant or irrelevant external stimuli)*
   6. *increase in goal-directed activity (at work, at school, or sexually) or psychomotor agitation*
   7. *excessive involvement in pleasurable activities that have a high potential for painful consequences (e.g., engaging in unrestrained buying sprees, sexual indiscretions, or foolish business investments)*

I'd been thinking about karma a lot recently. It was an unlikely word to lodge itself in my consciousness, given my lack of belief in anything supernatural. Although I'd gone through a "spiritual crisis" when I was young and naïve – a student in London, and had felt called to be a Lamb of God (that is a born-again, evangelical Christian), I'd subsequently, after a year or two of intense endeavour during which I'd almost packed everything up to become a missionary, become a dead-again atheist, or, as Ben calls me, because of my refusal to believe in anything that can't be physically proven, a 'radical empiricist.'

California, with its general air of irrational, tolerant kookiness, had been something of a test for me when I'd moved to San Francisco in the early nineties. I never got used to the way almost complete strangers would blurt out something intensely personal, or, even worse, friends who'd blurt out personal things about you in front of strangers thinking, hey, we're all Californians together, let's bare our souls. And those same friends, many of whom possessed qualities of intelligence and worldliness I otherwise esteemed, would constantly surprise me with their beliefs. For instance, after I told my friend Cecilia a sarcasm-laced tale about an abortive date with a cute hairdresser who'd turned me off as soon as he'd started talking about his encounter, in the Gulf of Mexico, with telepathic dolphins, Cecilia had looked at me quizzically, and had said, hesitantly, 'You mean you don't believe dolphins are telepathic?'

If you can picture me as a sort of extra tall Dana Scully, then Cecilia would be an unlikely feminine version of Fox Muldur. She's a sophisticated, intellectual woman, with dramatically high cheekbones, and elegantly coiffed, lightly graying hair, bilingual, brought up in Paris and Greece by a rather excitable Turkish mother, and a well-travelled father, who was a top U.S. diplomat. Like most glamorous lesbians, she's a gay-guy magnet, and I'd been drawn to her, as had many others. I'd frequently noticed her training people at the gym, and, after my first trainer had moved to Singapore, I'd walked up to Cecilia to ask her about training, drawn by her mysterious air and rather exotic features. (Her best friend Larry liked to imitate her, saying things like 'When the scent of myrrh wafts off the Bosporus ...'). Like all seekers at the spiritual smorgasbord, she harbours the idea that everybody else secretly believes likewise, and is just waiting to have somebody draw it out of them.

I'd hired Cecilia during the time when I had chronic fatigue syndrome and had needed to be pushed to work out (whereas now that I was in complete remission, I just paid her to be my friend.) One day, we were training at Market Street Gym in the Castro, and I began to grow unusually short of breath. Cecilia had me lie down on the bench, but I struggled even more to get my breath. I was on the edge of panic, and Cecilia hurried downstairs to get the manager. Abruptly, my body started to crawl with the sensation of pins and needles, and I felt that I was losing control of my muscles. I grabbed somebody and jerked out the words, feeling like such a drama queen, 'I need help'. I was rolled out of the gym in a wheelchair to the waiting ambulance, feeling very embarrassed at all the fuss. However, I staged a quick comeback and demurred on the trip to the hospital, and, instead, got Cecilia to drive me home, which was not necessarily the brightest idea given Cecilia's driving abilities, and her terror of driving my relatively large SUV. When we found my street blocked with a moving truck, Cecilia panicked, while I started to have another attack, and ran into my apartment to lie down, leaving Cecilia, who'd only just got her license, to attempt to parallel park the thing. The same ambulance crew that had come for me at the gym eventually reappeared to cart me to Davies emergency room. I was told that it was merely hyperventilation, but since I'd never experienced it before, I'd not recognized it. The Emergency Room gave me a Xanax and released me.

I went to bed that night with the phone on my bedside table in case I had another attack (ordinarily I switched the phone ringer off overnight). Strangely, the phone rang after ten. It was my practice to not answer the phone unless I recognized the number, so I ignored it. But when it rang again first thing in the morning, my intuition told me exactly what it was. My mother, who'd been sick for years, had died. When I compared the hour of her death with my attack of hyperventilation, it was, I must admit, convincingly

Broken Whole

contemporaneous, and Cecilia was incredulous that I couldn't accept it as anything other than coincidence.

I still don't believe in supernatural phenomena, but after the events that form the core of this book, I have to say I now consider myself a discretely spiritual person, albeit on my own resolute, highly personal terms. The first inkling of this development came during the early weeks of budding mania, with my experience of the concept of karma. I'd begun to develop homespun philosophies on this theme during the summer months when I'd begun to feel my depression recede. Ben likes to tell the story of, years ago, meeting an acquaintance of his best friend, Joe, in London, who'd described Ben as the single most outgoing person he'd ever met. He wasn't far from the truth. Ben can light up a room with his charm, and his almost endless selection (to other people at least, who haven't heard them twenty times) of dramatic stories told with excited (and loud) flair. At parties, you can often spot him in the centre of a group, gesturing animatedly and rather wildly with his hands, his voice clearly audible from downstairs, if not all the way down the street. His stories tend to get elaborated over time. For instance, last week, we were driving with out-of-town friends, and Ben was, as usual, holding forth with a story, this one from our trip to Budapest in 2008. I was sure our friends had heard it before, but were either too polite to say so, or had forgotten (which, at our age, is a frequent occurrence and probably a bit of a blessing.) And I had to keep chiming in with corrections to his description of trudging, with heavy luggage, up seven flights of stairs ('it was three'), to find our guest room furnished a la IKEA-1980 (he was right on that), and being molested by our tour-guide (who in fact merely rubbed a cold Pepsi can against his neck, and offered him a handful of condoms.)

I like to describe myself as an outgoing introvert, and, being with such a luminous partner, I've had to boost my own light so that it's visible, so to speak, from behind Ben's bushel. And after I started to recover from depression in the summer, I found it even easier to talk to people without any self-consciousness, and, feeling as if I was uncovering the real me for the first time, I too would hold forth at parties, with my own little circle gathered around me. I no longer felt that I had to fend for myself or risk being overshadowed by Ben. And I'd moved far from my old self-image of being a dorky, shy tall guy standing quietly in the corner, aloneness visible to all, possibly stashed there by a more extroverted partner. We felt as if we were well-liked as a couple, and that the energy we were giving out was being reflected back in abundance. In other words, it seemed we were the recipients of good karma.

The most vivid example of this sense of karma came when we got committed ... that is, joined ... or however you're supposed to describe the act of being brought together as one in a commitment ceremony. (The word *committed* has unhappy associations for me, given what was to happen less than two weeks after coming back from Dallas.) We were the first couple we knew to have such a ceremony, and we spent months planning it. On the day itself, we arrived at our house in a limousine at six in the evening, when everyone – one hundred people all told – had gathered in the tree-shaded lower garden beneath our house. A duet of *Bewitched* by Frank Sinatra and Patty LaBelle, belted out in the perfect late evening air, and, to the final chords, Ben and I approached the steps down to the garden. When we reached the edge of the patio, overlooking the garden below, it was the first time we'd seen the crowd: so many familiar faces turned our way. My brother Neil and his boyfriend Simon were there, along with one of Ben's sisters.

My dad had written a card to both of us, to be read out loud at the ceremony. The idea that my dad would one day give his blessings to my gay marriage would have struck me as ludicrous a decade earlier. To set the context, the minister briefly related my history with my father before reading the card aloud.

It had been hard to come out to my father, who had always placed such a high prize on masculinity. The first effort was a plan to tell him during a get together in Paris, after I'd moved to Philadelphia. But he'd forestalled me by telling me about the 'bunch of pansies' staying at his hotel. He'd added, 'We don't like Catholics, aren't fond of Jews, don't want to be around Pakis...' (a sort of catch all for anybody from South-East Asia) '... but the one thing we really can't stand is homosexuals!'

When I finally did come out to him, via the safer mode of the postal mail, when I was around twenty-three, it precipitated a period of over a decade where my sexuality was a forbidden and ignored subject between us. On one occasion, I'd mentioned – testing the water a little – going to a birthday party of a boyfriend of one of my good male friends, and, apparently, my dad was ill for a couple of weeks after that. But a couple of years after my mother died, by which time I'd fallen in love with Ben, I'd already regained some of my lost admiration for him due to the way he'd taken care of my dying mother, and I'd begun to call him weekly, as opposed to having semi-annual, forced phone conversations about football and politics. Initially, these more frequent calls were still about football and politics. But he had clearly changed by now. The experience of losing my mother had unveiled his inner emotional core, and he'd become sentimental and maudlin like many repressed Brits in old age, to an extent that made me uncomfortable. I was forever fearful he'd cry on the phone. In fact, I was the one who now clung desperately to the football and politics conversation, since it was a much safer playing field than feelings. This was all the height of irony, since it was such a role reversal: my discomfort with his expressiveness had its origin in his own severe reprobation of the softer emotions when I'd been a teenager. Now, I wondered, though: had he changed enough to be able to hear about Ben? I did feel stifled when talking to him, since I couldn't mention the most important thing in my life. Once again I chose the written word to tell him, saying, in closing, that I wouldn't push the issue; it was up to him to let me know if he wanted to continue the dialogue. When he wrote back, full of acceptance, he ended by saying that if Ben and I were half as happy as he'd been with my mother, then we'd be lucky indeed. Since I'd always seen their relationship as a model to aim for, this meant a lot to me, and brought an immediate rush of tears to my eyes. (Subsequently, on our first visit to London together as a couple, Ben was immediately accepted into the family. This was something of a mixed blessing, since my sisters have at least as many stories as Ben, and tell them with yet greater frequency, and, moreover, Ben also now had to bear the full brunt of the Adams' sense of humour.)

At our commitment ceremony, while my dad's card was being read, I looked around at people's faces, illuminated by candlelight in the dusk under the trees. I felt the acuteness of the moment, recalling, with a sense of wonderment, my journey from being a shy, awkward, working-class kid from a fishing town on the North Sea coast of England, to being here right now, marrying my boyfriend in front of a huge crowd of friends at our home in the Hollywood Hills. There were several sets of moist eyes, yet mine remained dry. I'd expected to cry, if at no other point than when I read my self-written vows aloud, but even now, my upbringing was speaking to me, bidding me to withhold open emotion.

The ceremony cemented our relationships with a relatively new group of friends, all of whom, apparently, had been talking for weeks about our ceremony. I'd never expected, especially since I was full of the San Francisco prejudice against all things LA, that when I moved to Los Angeles I'd end up with the best circle of friends I'd ever had, many of them gay couples of long standing. It was, we felt, karma in action.

Ben maintains that I rarely do things by half measures. After I came back from Dallas, this was certainly the case with karma, which was soon to become ... Karma WeHo, the West Hollywood superclub. Even before Dallas, the karma concept had begun fascinating me, and while we were in San Diego for gay pride, I'd thought of getting a karma tattoo on my chest. (Just as well that I didn't: getting a tattoo while manic is probably at least as foolish as getting tattooed while intoxicated.) I spoke to Ben about replacing Brewster, our beautiful Bernese mountain dog who'd recently died, with a little dog called Karma (so that I could have karma with me all the time.) I went so far as to apply for the CA vanity license plate KARMA-X. When I got notice of its approval, months later, I was well over the whole idea of karma (and Karma), and Ben, certainly, would never want to hear that word again. Besides, you're probably asking for trouble by driving a Land Rover around LA with a KARMA-X license plate.

After coming back from Dallas, finding not only did I still have a job but was eligible to go on short-term disability, I felt I had license to devote myself full-time to the Karma idea. I began to assemble an outlandishly ambitious business proposal, which I emailed to friends whom I was considering as potential partners, inviting them to an evening meeting at a bar/restaurant called O-Bar, on Thursday night. It was my stated goal to be ready to meet with a VP I knew at Bank of America, on Friday, to start the process of getting venture funding.

Looking back, I have to say that my friends reacted with astonishing grace. It must have seemed very strange that, out of the blue, I would push forwards so insistently on something of such magnitude having absolutely no background in either business or entertainment. It was only later that I realized they were all secretly worried about my behaviour. But, at the time, I had such ardour and self-confidence that I either didn't hear, or brushed aside any notes of doubt that were expressed.

At the same time, I'd introduced another source of complexity into my life. On the Monday after I returned from Dallas, absurdly worried that somehow my company would reach through the Internet and capture and erase all the non-work related information on my laptop, I set about separating my work and personal lives completely, getting a new laptop, removing all my personal emails and documents from my work laptop, and buying, with Ben's generous financial assistance, every piece of hardware and software I could conceivably need. I rushed headily about the UCLA computer store, accumulating gadgets and software packages, while Ben looked on with helpless concern.

Over the weekend, it had seemed extremely urgent to take this step since I believed it would be possible I'd be fired. But now that this no longer seemed at all likely, I still retained a sense of extreme urgency, driving myself to get everything set up and working on my new laptop. The same sort of complexity that had dogged me in Dallas kept reappearing. I could suddenly no longer receive email at my new email-address, the address of which I'd sent out to everybody I knew just the day before. I worked until late into the night, every night, on hold to technical support lines, becoming furious at the incompetence of the people on the other end of the phone-line. Ben didn't say anything, but he couldn't understand why it was so important to get everything working at once. And neither can I, looking back. Yet I also now recognize that it was part of the radically shifted perspective of mania. Ben volunteered to sleep downstairs so that I wouldn't have to worry about waking him once I'd finished on the computer late each night.

By Wednesday, after insuperable problems with my original choice for a domain host, Infinology (who turned out to be scam artists), I had to give up on my new email address, and set up a temporary hotmail email address instead. It was embarrassing to have to tell my friends that I was changing my email address once again. (And this wouldn't be the last time.)

My biggest frustration was with customer-service operations. I'd call and have to navigate through a long computer menu, only to be kept on hold. If I got a real, live person then they wouldn't be able to answer my question, and they'd reroute me to a different person. After listening to them tell me how to navigate an operating system I knew better than they did, they'd arrive – after consulting their script – at the ultimate solution to the problem, requiring to uninstall and reinstall the software, switch off my firewall, and disable all the other add-ons I'd patiently installed, expecting I'd be satisfied just to get their one piece working. I lost my temper frequently, and would yell withering, articulate put-downs at the hapless customer-support people, who either refused to entertain my ideas for improving their process, or simply couldn't understand why I'd even be suggesting changes.

It was the same syndrome that had bugged me in Dallas, and was the origin of an idea that wouldn't fully bloom until the apex of the crisis, but which led directly to the name of this book. My laptop was becoming so complex that it was taking ten minutes just to reboot. Complexity was making it impossible for me to do even basic things like sending email. Didn't software designers realize that there had to be a limit to complexity before things became unusable? Complexity was the antithesis of completeness – or wholeness.

Just as in Dallas, however, I was beginning to realize that I'd brought this on myself once more. In my quiet moments, I'd wonder why I really needed all the stuff I'd bought. A more important question that I failed to ask myself, was, why was I working seventeen hour days on installing my new laptop?

The work on the laptop wasn't even the prime mover of the week. That place was reserved for Club Karma. As with the laptop, everything became inconceivably urgent. I had to have our meeting at O-Bar come what may, that first Thursday after Dallas, and I spent a day running around West Hollywood and Beverly Hills, getting business cards printed, and a beautiful, professional-looking business-plan made. Obstacles kept getting thrown in my path: I left my ATM card in a machine at the bank, and got blisteringly mad – almost raving – when they told me they couldn't mail it to me. I charged off, only to realize hours later, that I'd left my driver's license behind, at the bank. I only came across the missing driver's license when, enraged at a forty-five minute wait time on Bank of America's customer-service line, I tried to start up a new bank account at City National Bank, intending to transfer everything to them. Needless to say, I didn't get very far without my driver's license. Losing my credit-cards and driver's license was to become a repeated (and dangerous) motif in the upcoming week or so.

Meanwhile, FedEx had lost my order for business cards, and couldn't turn around a new order in time for the meeting that night. I had a copy of the design on a flash-drive, but they weren't allowed to use external flash-drives, and this gave me the pretext to throw another tantrum. I was becoming almost a parody of the self-entitled Los Angeleno. And, in everything I did, complexity and self-imposed pressure were my own enemies, the same unquestioning drive that had thrust me into taking on too much in Dallas.

By the time of the meeting at O-Bar, I was ready. But, to my dismay, I started getting calls from my friends that they couldn't make it. They offered a variety of excuses, and I took them in my stride, not reflecting, for a moment, that my hyper-charged impetuosity was scaring them off.

My mind was spouting with other ideas, and I felt as if my intelligence was expanding geometrically. Indeed, to this day, I maintain that if my IQ had been measured while I was in the midst of high mania, it would have been off the charts. There is something about the disorder that lights up parts of your brain that are otherwise shrouded in shadows. Yet I didn't know that I was manic. Instead, I thought I'd somehow tapped into astounding intellectual growth. In the isolation of an elevator I would say aloud the mantra I'd been repeating to myself for a while (and which is now hard to admit on paper): that I was the most intelligent person who'd ever lived.

The Polymath

My efforts at creativity were branching out in many different directions simultaneously. I started a blog in which I rambled in an incredibly grandiose, stream-of-consciousness fashion. I'm ashamed to say that my first blog entry was subtitled: *The Blog Heard Around the World*; it was so profound, I thought, that there might be news cameras outside my door in the morning. I emailed it to everybody I knew, and, for some of them, this was the first they knew about the *new* me. Amazingly, Ben didn't at that moment whip out the DSM IV manual and shove the definition of mania down my throat.

> *Quite where to start almost defeats me. How does one grow morally from a pygmy to a behemoth in the space of a week? Is it possible to expand in the physical, moral, intellectual and emotional realms but not the spiritual? I've been absorbing a million ideas daily, and since I've always been driven to catalogue my thoughts, and have always had a lot of ideas, with an interest in organizing them, I'm naturally trying to process the information flowing through my mind. But what happens if the information flow is so great that it's beyond me? Is it possible that there could be just too much information for me to control, and that I'll be driven anyway to somehow encompass it, because of my pesky refusal to be beaten up by my own ideas?*

(I couldn't realize how prophetically I was speaking.)

> *No; the answer is 'no'. In fact, I was almost wrung dry in Dallas. But I saved every madman's scribble, some of which will dribble onto this page, at a pace not inconsiderable, given time.*

Now I'd like to talk about Star Trek, and in particular Leonard Nimoy. I always identified with both the actor (a dignified man with intellect, charisma and warmth - in short, a mensch) and his character. As a kid, I used to dream I'd wake up and somehow discover I was Mr. Spock. Not that I was anywhere as substantial a person at any time in my life.

But I'm thinking of what happened to him in Star Trek: The Motion Picture as, drawn by his personal needs, he strove to make his mind complete by melding with Vejur, the machine that had learned all that was knowable. He strove to master the ideas, but in the end even he could not wrestle them to a stand-still. And through that he became both more human, and more powerful (emotionally, intellectually and morally) than he'd ever anticipated. So my story comes full circle. Mr. Spock becomes Leonard Nimoy. And skinny Keith Adams, the moral pygmy, became Keith Adams the ... what? Where is his ship heading?

In addition to my off-the-cuff blog entries, and starting a column on a local gay website, wehonews.com, I bought the domain-name ideas-network.net with the intention, someday, of starting up a *Wikipedia* for ideas; I thought I might become a DJ and bought some DJ software; I continued work on my book while planning a second on the subject of genius; and formulated an outline for a new short movie to shoot. Even at home, I was untiring: stripping the varnish off an elaborate set of shelves to repaint it black and grey; buying a ton of lumber to convert our king-size bed into a platform bed (not put off by my complete lack of experience in carpentry); and reupholstering our day bed (in a fetching white fur material with large black dots, making the finished item look like a dead cow.)

Broken Whole

Apart from the club, Karma, into which I poured most of my creative ideas, I thought about the book. I felt that the story I had to tell - of how a damaged man recovers his full potential – was compelling. I'd need a literary agent and perhaps somebody to ghost-write it for me, since I believed I wouldn't have the time (which was clearly true, in view of having to reupholster our day bed, become a DJ, and start a cruise-line. I'm joking about the cruise-line.)

I began to seek publicity so that I could further my ideas. I sent sexy, glossy photos, along with a biography, to all the local gay magazines, thinking they'd be interested in a story like mine, particularly since I was going to be opening a gay club. I made an appointment with a PR firm, and met there with a woman with the unlikely name of Sparkle. She showed great interest and excitement in my ideas, and we discussed a contract of $5,000 to get my name, and story out there into the press. After the initial meeting, I never heard from her, and she didn't return my calls. I ascribed her lack of response to an attitude with which I was becoming increasingly familiar: you're nobody in Los Angeles, unless you have the right connections; or unless, of course, you're already a celebrity.

I found I had a huge amount of energy to put into my workouts now. I was lifting heavier and heavier weights. And I ceased to care what people thought about my clothes, believing I could wear anything I wanted, pulling it off with charm and self-confidence. I felt I was on the verge of huge changes in my life; that I'd become well-known, and would have to look good for business meetings. So I made sure I had a spray-tan at all times, and that my hair was styled regularly into a highlighted faux-maux. I started to use beauty products regularly for the first time. Wherever I went, I met and engaged people with unashamed confidence in my identity. I had, no longer, any shame; had nothing to hide. People seemed drawn to me, just as I, having always had a need to connect, was drawn to others. Under no circumstances was I afraid to make eye contact or start up a conversation. And I never had any doubts about what to say. Nothing held my humour and self-confidence in check. I knew myself through and through; the world was opening up for me, and I could contain it all in my hands without losing my values.

Book III – Chaos - Two Weeks in August
The Path Towards the Summit

In the weeks leading up to the first inklings of mania, I'd observed that my ease at talking to people when clubbing had leached over into my daily life. This was confirmed in the work week in Dallas that immediately followed; I felt that I could speak to anybody and instantly charm them, or in a business setting, win them over to my point of view. During the week after I came back from Dallas, our cleaning maids brought a young niece with them, and I wasn't particularly surprised that for the first time in my life I could even talk to children.

Things changed with Ben too. Back during the first honeymoon year of our relationship, Ben thought he'd snagged an über romantic guy; the sort of guy who'd write him love poems. Once, when on business in New York, I missed him so acutely that I cried after I wrote and sent him one of my poems. It's hard to believe now that I wasn't surprised by the person I became during those heady months after we fell in love. What was disappointing to Ben is that the old Keith stole back upon me about a year into our relationship, the Keith who'd learned that affectionate emotions were a sign of weakness, and who'd buried them so deeply that they weren't even detectable at a subterranean level. I couldn't even bring myself to sign off emails or text messages with "Hugs" to my closest friend, and I'd ceased to find it comfortable to call Ben "baby", even by text-message.

Now, however, for the first time in my life, I felt truly whole. All of the mental energy I'd previously deployed in self-consciousness, introspection, keeping emotion at bay, and even in self pity: all of that energy was now freed up. I felt that I could afford to give from my riches, and it enabled me both to be more vulnerable with Ben, as well as more caring, loving and empathic. When I held Ben in my arms each night, I felt strong, protective, and wise.

One unexpected effect of my emotional strength was that many physical ailments disappeared. For the whole of my thirties I had had painful tendonitis in my left wrist. I had been unable to type for more than a couple of hours without pain. In Dallas, however, and then again in the following week, where I was setting up my new laptop, I could now work seventeen hour days with no pain at all.

Both Ben and my therapist were worried that I might be hypomanic (a less severe form of mania that can, however, develop into the real thing.) I didn't agree, but consented nonetheless to go on Depakote, a mood stabilizer, to pacify their worries. Although I understood Ben's fears as valid, given his experience with his previous bipolar boyfriend, I felt he was being overly anxious: couldn't he happily accept that I'd simply inherited my full potential?

In the middle of the week after I came back from Dallas, there was an event at I-candy in West Hollywood, to find new cover models for a Las Vegas gay magazine called Envy. Dean's beautiful ex-boyfriend, Stan, and I made plans to go together.

It's always been inescapable, due to my height, that I'll be noticed when I walk into a bar. For most of my life it was a curse. But tonight I felt – or assumed – everybody was looking at me and seeing the self-image I was carrying around in my head. Within a few minutes of entering, I'd already been photographed, and had met the publisher of the magazine. 'You're it,' he said. (Of course, I never heard from him again.)

Ben's birthday was approaching and it seemed to me to be the perfect opportunity to have a large party that would simultaneously promote Karma. I was meeting so many people that I could easily see us having two-hundred guests. Ben was dismayed at the idea, but I convinced him to agree to half that number.

Broken Whole

I'm sure all our friends had registered the huge shift in my emotional energy. We'd meet them at the Abbey, our favourite bar in West Hollywood, and I'd dress and talk with an ease I'm sure they'd never seen. In fact, I'd become more Ben-like than ever. And I was aware, now and then, although none of them said anything, that they looked at me with outwardly amused but slightly wary perplexity.

I was working on my various projects until late at night, and Ben was still sleeping downstairs so that he wouldn't disturb me. By the time I'd go to bed, my mind would be racing so fast I'd need a huge swig of vodka and a Xanax to knock me out. My creative fervour and late working nights were driving Ben crazy with worry, and his worry was making me angry and irritable. I found myself continually suppressing my ideas and insights in order to avoid inflaming his anxiety. But sometimes I'd vent my frustration in a show of fury that I'd instantly regret and apologize for.

I felt like a fundamentally changed person. Nothing got to me any more except incompetence. No, that's not completely true. My patience, always scarce to begin with, was also limited with respect to what I saw as the tendency – on the part of both Ben and David – to interpret everything I said as evidence I was manic. I'd argue that there were many extraordinary people – Bill Clinton, for instance – who never got labelled as manic. Bill Clinton had had the good fortune to understand who he was, and what he was capable of, whereas my own journey of self-discovery had been cut short by depression, shyness and chronic fatigue. Unsurprisingly, the comparison to Bill Clinton did not help my case, with Ben and David, for not being manic.

The alternative to talking about my ideas was to not talk at all, so I'd tell myself to shut up. If this change was real and not manic, then sooner or later my ideas would speak for themselves. Yet communication - being understood, and feeling connected - these things had always been of utmost importance to me, so it was all but impossible for me to stop talking.

The Idea that Would Change the World, 2nd week of August

I was working at home, as usual, wrestling with getting my new laptop fully installed. And, borne of hours of frustration, I came up with a seemingly flawless idea. Throughout the week, I'd spent ten hours daily on the phone trying and (mostly) failing to make progress with intractable problems; endless phone menus, lack of human response, and inadequately trained employees with very strong Indian accents who'd say things like 'I'm very pleased to be offering you the excellent service today, sir.'

On this morning, my patience reached a breaking point. I'd bought antivirus software from Symantec, and to fully install it, I needed a confirmation code, which was supposed to be in an email. I never received the email, and after an hour poking around on their website, I'd not even been able to find a customer-service number.

That's when a light-bulb went off. On the search engine AltaVista you can restrict your search to pages within a single domain, for example, Symantec.com. So the first part of my strategy was to find the name of a very senior officer at Symantec. I expected that the search would be relatively easy to find in press releases, looking for phrases like "vice-president".

Then I did a similar search, this time for the name and phone number of a customer-service manager, again expecting to find this in press releases. Even if I didn't get the phone number, I could call the main switchboard and ask for the person by name.

With the information ready, I called Symantec and asked, in my best, diffident British accent, to speak to the customer-service manager whose name I'd found. I reached his administrative assistant.

'I'm a personal friend of your Senior VP for Development,' I said. 'I'm in a rather uncomfortable situation. I'm a senior editor for technology at the New York

Times, and I'm writing a comparative review of antivirus software. I've had considerable trouble getting your software to work. But, you know, since your senior VP is my friend, I'd rather not embarrass him by writing a bad review. Would it be possible for somebody to call me to help me through my problem?'

After I was through with Symantec, it began to dawn on me that if everybody used this simple approach to bypass the immense mechanisms that companies had put in place to keep customers at a distance, then those companies would have to scramble to reinvent their systems. For some reason which eludes me now, I believed this would have a global economic effect. The fragile ropes tethering my sense-of-reality to the ground were beginning to fray.

Grandiosity is the hallmark of mania. I thought that I was brilliant and destined for fame and riches beyond my imagination. This was the moment where the kindling sparks of mania turned into a voracious firestorm tearing through my brain. With each passing second after coming up with this idea, my manic brain visualised greater and greater possibilities, each of them further removed from reality than the last. I thought that I would never again have to work. I was feeling, moment by moment, increasingly freed from all the urges that had been driving me all week, as my mind surveyed the likely outcomes of my discovery. I realized I would probably never use the laptop I'd fevered over all week. In fact, I might never have to use a computer again, since I'd have people to do that for me. So I decided to relax for the first time since returning from Dallas. I could spend the day indulging myself. I dressed to kill, and left the house floating through the gates towards a princely future, leaving the house unlocked, and taking with me only the car keys. It would be fun to see if, despite not having cash, my ATM card, or driver's license with me (the latter two which still resided at the Bank of America on the Sunset Strip), charm and intelligence alone could get me through a day of pampering. At that moment I truly thought I might never need to come back to our house again, since by the end of the day I'd be sure of being immensely rich.

I decided to start by renting an expensive car with a driver, to have myself driven to a spa for a massage. I called a Beverly Hills rental car agency (which I'd used, without telling Ben, the previous week, when I'd felt that our second car – my previously beloved solar yellow, seven-year old Nissan Xterra – was inappropriate to my business aims) to drive over to me, at Starbucks, the most expensive car they had available, thinking I would perhaps get a Bentley. (Instead, I had to settle for a high-end Lexus.)

While I was waiting, I walked next door to buy a new cell-phone from Cingular. I already had a cellular-plan with T-Mobile, so I can't immediately summon up any explanation for why I'd left my cell phone at home, other than doing it for fun, and the challenge to see what I could accomplish without money and identification.

In a manic episode you lose sight of priorities. Since I needed to get back to Starbucks in time for the arrival of the rental car, I couldn't afford to spend much time in Cingular getting the new phone, which I was, by the by, trying to get without identification or a credit card. I found myself seething over every obstacle, and I browbeat the staff mercilessly. The truly astonishing thing about my behaviour was that as soon as I got what I wanted, all my fury disappeared, and I became calm, genial and relaxed, as if nothing had happened. If I could have seen my behaviour in the cell-phone store from outside myself, even without knowing that there was truly nothing urgent about getting a new cell-phone, or that I had a perfectly good one at home, I'd have been repelled. This cell-phone, moreover, was to have a very short life. In fact, in the late afternoon, I'd throw it, along with my watch, into a parking lot as I tried to slow my raging mind on my blazing path across Hollywood, to make the couples' counselling meeting with Ben.

When I returned to Starbucks, there was no sign of the car. But it didn't matter because I still had to find a driver.

Broken Whole

Just at that moment, Darryl, a charismatic, imposing, dignified black actor friend of mine appeared and I asked him, insultingly I now realize with regret, if he'd consider driving me around for the day for a couple of hundred dollars. He said he couldn't because he had an acting class to make. I told him that if he played his cards right he'd never have to take another acting class again. I was thinking I could make all my friends rich too. Instead of telling me that I was crazy, he humoured me, smiled, and went inside Starbucks to get some coffee.

He was inside only a very few minutes, but it was long enough for me to stage what I thought was a remarkable demonstration. Darryl came out of Starbucks and sat beside me, and I told him that I could predict the future. He asked me what was going to happen next. I looked around, and spotted a young man in a pink t-shirt, across the street. 'In a few moments,' I told him, 'that man is going to come over and ask you if you're an actor, and where can he take acting lessons.'

After a couple of minutes, the young man crossed the road and approached us. 'Excuse me,' he stammered, 'are you actors?'

'Why do you want to know? ' I pointed at Darryl to signify he was the actor.

'I'm trying to find out where I can get acting lessons,' he responded.

From my point of view, the incident proved to me how easy it was, if you had a facile way with people, to control them into both doing what you wanted, and seeing what you wanted them to see. What had happened was that the moment Darryl had gone into Starbucks, the young man had approached, while I was sitting there basking in my own limelight, and had asked me about acting lessons. In a split second, I'd dreamed up my little plan to startle Darryl, and had hustled the kid across the road, telling him to come back when my friend joined us. (Manic people are often capable of great improvisation, and general linguistic legerdemain, deploying, sometimes unconsciously, devices such as alliteration and onomatopoeia.)

Darryl was good-humouredly but nonetheless stubbornly unimpressed with my performance, and would still not agree to be my driver. So I called the store across the street to speak to the manager, one of the many people with whom I'd recently become friendly, and asked him if he could spare one of his employees to drive me for an hour or two. When he wasn't immediately responsive, I once again completely misplaced my own sense of priorities, and lied to him that it was a life-threatening situation.

All of the self-imposed complications had eaten into the day and it was already mid-afternoon by the time I acquired my driver, a tall, amiable guy named Myles. And I was exhausted. Since I hadn't yet acquired my riches, I decided that trying to charm my way into a hotel was beyond even my new abilities, and I asked Miles just to drive me home and drop me off, and then return the car to the agency for me.

During that ride home, my mind truly escaped its moorings, and I started to talk to Myles in tones of manic brilliance. It seemed to me that my intellect was expanding at the speed of light; that the universe was unfolding for me, in all its complexity. I was flooded with incredible ideas. I talked unrelentingly about do-it-yourself philosophies which sprang into existence as needed, when I merely glanced in their direction, fastening on the nature of reality.

'How do we know for sure that there is anything out there beyond the movie screen playing in our mind?'

Myles didn't have an answer. I looked around at all the plants by the roadside, so intricate and detailed, then cast my eyes over the enormous view of Los Angeles you get coming down Mulholland towards the 101.

'What if everything we see is actually just constructed by my mind when I need it? It's unlikely, I know. I mean, I've driven this drive hundreds of times, and all the details seem correct. But what if some plant has swapped places, or a building has leaped across the road? Would I even notice?'

I didn't really need Myles to respond.

'You know, it's actually physically possible,' I tossed at him, in an aside, 'according to quantum theory, that a building could spontaneously dissolve and reassemble somewhere else. It's just that you'd have to wait several times the length of the existence of the universe to see it since it's so vanishingly unlikely.'

I looked at him to see how that thought struck him.

'I know what you're thinking. That it's far more plausible to believe that everything is exactly the same as yesterday. And it's because it's real. And I agree - it doesn't seem possible that my mind could reconstruct all this detail every time I make this drive.'

As we drove further (I suppose I should say 'as I perceived myself driving further' but let's try to keep this simple), I came up with the idea that maybe the mind is powered by an enormous computer. Maybe the universe really does exist in some form, but we ourselves are incorporeal.

'So what,' I asked a subdued Myles, 'if I - or you for that matter - was/were the only mind? You'd have no way of knowing for sure: the computer could be mocking up all your friends and family right along with the Los Angeles cityscape and the daisies.'

'You're probably thinking - Ha! You're (Keith) speaking, and I'm listening, and I can even respond if I want. That is, you, Myles, can respond to what Keith is saying. And Keith sees Myles listening. Therefore we must both exist. But I could be having the perception of your existence, when in fact you're just part of my constructed reality. And you could experience the reality of listening to something your constructed reality tells you is coming from another person. Either way, it's possible there's just one of us. And it's impossible for the one who's real to know that the other isn't.'

My mind was taking leaps into the unknown. I now know that in reality, none of this is either as profound or original as I then believed. Back them, I'd never have been able to imagine I wasn't having startlingly original thoughts, or, at the least, that the computer could conjure up the perception that somebody else had thought along these lines.

'Okay, granted that a computer capable of making up and reconstructing such immense experiences - the night sky for example, or watching a symphony being performed live – would have to be incredibly powerful. It would have to be an artificial reality generator, required to model the entire universe in real time, in utterly convincing detail. The only way that I can imagine the possibility of such a computer is to think on universal scales. What if the universe itself is a gigantic quantum computer designed to manufacture my (or your) reality? '

Another tangent occurred to me. 'Wouldn't that mean that you and the universe are one?'

The very next second, though, I had a new idea.

'Actually, ' I said, thinking myself inconceivably compelling, 'the only thing that this computer has to construct is your perception of the current Now - everything you're feeling, seeing, hearing, touching, smelling at this moment. That requires a lot less computing power, since everything you're not experiencing right now does not need to be calculated. It just needs, for example, to focus on the car, and the street to either side. Oh, and, I guess,' I said modestly, 'my conversation.'

'Hmm, but what about the past ... and memory? You might say that you remember what you did an hour ago, and everything since an hour ago, and it all seems like one seamless whole. You met this crazy guy who wanted you to drive him around for the day, right?'

'Also, I guess, if I turn my head rapidly, I see just what I expect to see. If I run up a hill quickly, the view is what I envisioned from down below. And if I see somebody I haven't seen in years, I might say they hadn't changed a bit, but really I'd recognize the signs of ageing'.

I was on a roll, almost unstoppable.

'If each *Now* is an island unto itself, then the only thing telling me what was in the previous *Nows* is my memory. And that memory may also be an artifact of the Now, constructed at need. In other words, for each *Now*, the computer manufactures all of your perceptions, including your perceptions of your memories. Your actual perceived reality may be violently different from second to second, yet the computer tells your memory that it's seen each fresh scene before. This makes its task even easier. All it has to do is make something up for your senses, make something else up for your memory, and tie the two together so that you experience continuity.'

'God, I mean, if it's all true, then what does it mean that I can be currently in a Now where I'm speaking about the nature and reality of the *Now*? It's layers upon layers, I'm telling you.'

I suddenly thought of the implications of the so called *Multiverse* on my theory, an idea which could have easily given me another thirty minutes, but I decided it was time to give Myles a rest; and, besides: I wondered what he was thinking. I looked expectantly at him; he hadn't spoken now in ten minutes.

'What brand is your belt? It's really cool,' Myles asked.

I laughed. 'J. Lindberg. You know, Myles, it's karma that you're my driver today. Anybody else would likely have crashed the car after hearing all that. But you're grounded. You're probably the only person who could have safely driven me home.'

As we rounded the bend onto Cahuenga, for the last part of the trip, I found myself wondering about the lack of expansion in the spiritual realm: after all, I felt I'd expanded in the physical, emotional, intellectual and moral dimensions so rapidly, shouldn't the spiritual open to me also? And instantly, I literally had the sensation of the sea floor opening, with a deep subterranean rumble, a massive rift through which a blinding white light emerged, and I began to understand God. I had the most startling series of thoughts so far, quite scary even to myself as I thought through the consequences. But just before I could start up another discourse, my cell phone rang, and it was a tearful Ben, wondering where I was; why hadn't I shown up for couples' counselling? I immediately asked Myles to turn the car around to head back through Hollywood, and, after we ran into insurmountable traffic, I took off on foot, my head wrestling at the same time with cosmic theories and the urgent need to keep Ben from worrying about me.

This was the moment that precipitated the crisis I wrote about earlier in this book, in the opening chapter, the day I almost went insane. As I'd predicted in *The Blog Heard Around the World*, I was to have my Spock-melding-with-Vejur moment on the streets of Hollywood.

Unleashed, mid August

The week after I had my *encounter with the void* (as told in the Prelude of this book) was surprisingly normal. There was definitely some repair work going on, but we kept our focus on each other, and chose activities that made both of us happy. However, I found myself continuing to hide things from Ben to avoid worrying him, despite having nearly gone insane while trying to protect him from hurt.

I continued to believe I was on the edge of fulfilling my birth-right as a gifted, creative person, and it was a struggle to keep Ben's trust. From my point of view, yes, I'd almost gone crazy on Friday, but it had been worry for Ben that had driven me there; it didn't mean I was manic. For the most part, we tried not to talk about it.

As the week progressed, I started to get more and more enthusiastic about Club Karma. We had our couple's therapy session on Wednesday with Paul, and as I drove there to meet Ben, I called him preemptively, and told him that I could no longer carry his worries for him. They were mostly irrational, I said, so I would no longer get anxious over, for instance, what he thought about my club ideas, or my spending. This was met with silence initially, but when we were in the waiting room at Paul's, Ben reached over and took my hand and said that what I'd said was valid.

I was finally off the leash, dangerously so: free to pursue my goals effectively unsupervised, and, since I was on leave from work, I had plenty of time in which to do this. I was convinced that we would never again need to worry about money. If the club didn't pan out, then there was always customerserviceanytime.com, the new name for my dream that could change the world. And if neither of those worked out, I'd start a computer consulting firm, while working to finish my book. I was so divorced from reality that I simply couldn't imagine a scenario where we wouldn't enjoy a flood of new income in the coming weeks and months.

It's one of the mysteries of adulthood: why you can see in yourself so many traits learned from your parents, yet miss a few crucial ones. In my case, I had my dad's attraction for beauty, curiosity, and love of books, as well as his passion to set things right. I learned moral values and manners, and their importance, from both my parents. But I was totally failing in my dad's tradition of managing money. Although he had had a white-collar management job, my dad surely never made much more than a quarter of what I was making. Yet with that income he raised four children and bought a house.

Perhaps we only follow those things in our parents we don't resent. And since all of my friends in high school had more money than we did, I suppose I couldn't wait to make some money of my own in order to spend it. From college through graduate school, I made a habit of balancing my check book. But sometime in my twenties, I got bored even with that, and ever since then, I'd had almost no savings. I didn't even start building a 401k until my mid-thirties. (Even right now, towards the end of the month, I have only about a thousand dollars to my name, including savings. The reason why I'm in bad financial straits will become apparent in the next paragraph.)

So I didn't have a good financial history to begin with. Now, when I believed I'd soon be rich, I spread money around with inconceivable abandon. I spent thousands on infrastructure for my various web ventures. And I acquired new credit and store cards, indulging my weakness for clothes and accessories, with the excuse that I'd need to look good for business and social meetings. I became a regular in Beverly Hills, at Barneys New York, Saks Fifth Avenue, Neimann Marcus and D & G. I'd blaze through the Beverly Center, eyes afire with a consumptive gleam matched only by the dollar signs lighting up the eyes of the sales people, who now greeted me by name.

I bought a Diesel leather laptop bag, which proved too small; so I spent almost a thousand dollars on a gorgeous Italian leather bag whose outside flap was covered with fur.

Broken Whole

(It too would prove inadequate to carry my heavy laptop.) Next there was a two-thousand Gucci leather jacket from Neiman Marcus, which had to be tailored to fit. In fact, the tailor said that what I wanted – the sleeves lengthening – couldn't be done, at least elegantly. But to my mind, there was a solution to every problem. 'Take the sleeves off, and add leather, cut from the inside, at the top of the sleeve,' I said. It's an illustration that mania truly can inspire unusual creative thoughts that, in this case, not even the expert Italian tailor had considered.

Luggage from both Prada and D & G soon followed, along with J. Lindberg shirts, D&G jeans, a Vuitton toiletries bag, a Ferragamo clutch, a tiny little Montblanc notebook-wallet and pen, a Paul Smith credit-card wallet, an extraordinarily blingy five-hundred dollar key-chain by Alexander McQueen (a thick bronze chain with an eight-inch bronze articulated skeleton dangling at one end), and yet another key chain from D&G, and two Bluetooth headsets – one of them hot pink, to go with my new Motorola cell-phone. (I got into pink for a while, and sheathed my new Sony laptop with a shiny pink cover.) Oh, and I bought a Treo too, but didn't realize it would only work on a different cellular network than the one I was on. The only one of these purchases that truly made sense, given my penchant for note-taking, was the Montblanc wallet, although I will admit that I consider the Gucci jacket one of the best fruit of mania, and adore it sinfully. I've spent most of my life without a well-fitting casual coat, since coats just seem to come in one shape, so that if you have extraordinarily long arms, you're presumed to also have enormous girth.

As I spent, I met people, inevitably. Apart from deliberately connecting with people who might become part of my club experience, such as a couple of well-known DJs, I'd encounter random, interesting people wherever I went. Strangers had no reason to believe I was manic, because they had nothing to compare me against, having not met me before. I'd storm into a store and hold court with sales associates and well-heeled shoppers. They'd ask me what I did, and I'd tell them about the club I was planning to open, Karma, and we'd exchange business cards. When I opened new store-card accounts, I'd describe my occupation as "polymath".

I was also meeting, in great numbers, young, gorgeous men. We'd strike up a conversation as I shopped for socks, say, in LASC in West Hollywood. I'd be unintimidated by their supermodel looks. Seeking potential models for promotional materials for my club, I'd tell them about Karma, and proffer the business card.

I wonder now how accurate my self-perception was. I believed that I was cutting a figure. I was energetic without restraint, had no self doubt, and unlimited self-confidence. I thought myself striking, engaging, enthusiastic, exciting … and many other words ending in "ing". People seemed to respond to me as though they echoed my self-perception. But I now know that mania makes you subject to cognitive errors and misapprehensions. Ideas that might seem either crazy or ordinary when in a normal frame of mind can seem brilliant and original when manic. One day in Barneys, in Beverly Hills, I was trying on an exotic, fur-lined vest in a public area of the fitting room, and had both the sales associate and tailor fussing over my exacting demands for a perfect, body-hugging fit. While I had my hands out to either side as the tailor was measuring me, I struck up a conversation with a man who turned out to be a major menswear designer. He seemed interested in my club idea, and I told him I'd invite him to the opening of Karma, when it got off the ground. I jokingly asked him if they were looking for models, and he gave me his business card. What did this man see? Did he see what I felt I was projecting? Or was he humouring somebody who he thought might be slightly crazy? How often, in situations like that, were people just putting up a front of being interested while wondering inside when is this guy going to shut up?

Broken Whole

As I left Barneys after this particular encounter, I remembered, with some amusement, a quite different interaction with a celebrity a year earlier at the Paul Smith store on Melrose Avenue. I was in a bad depression, and, having no work project to occupy my time, I was trying to get a gay-wedding-planning business off the ground. (This idea seemed so *not me*. Ben had suggested it based on the success of our commitment ceremony, which I'd largely organized. I envision a wedding planner as being smooth, almost certainly fey, good with women, and pushy, all attributes which didn't fit with my then self-image as a masculine man who'd have to play a role in order to overcome the lack of self-belief instilled by depression.) An older gay man was eyeing me, while waiting for a female friend of his who was talking to somebody behind my left shoulder. As he stared, I did my best to ignore him, but then I started to recognize the voice of his friend, and, looking at her out of the corner of my eye, I realized, sure enough, it was Ellen DeGeneres. Such a wasted opportunity, I'd thought to myself at the time. (This was, of course, before I'd discovered the concept of karma.) If I'd have talked to the older guy, I could have met Ellen, and could have given her my wedding-planning business card. On the other hand, if I'd been in my current frame of mind, I'd have not even needed to go through her male friend; I would have walked right up to her and introduced myself, and invited her, of course, to the opening of Karma. I may even have been bold enough to ask her to do a show about me, along the lines of the idea I'd pitched to a Bravo Channel executive I met at Starbucks this week.

With my plans for Karma gaining such inevitable strength, and at the rate I was meeting new people, I had now begun to recalibrate my goals. It was astounding to me to recognize how far I'd come in so short a time. In short order, I'd permanently defeated any doubts about my body; had indeed learned to use it as an asset. For a while thereafter, the seemingly unstoppable growth in my intellect had held me in thrall. Yet now, just days later, I was realizing that the greatest gift of all lay in my self-confidence borne out of the other new traits. It was my unshakable self-belief, and the emotional intelligence I seemed to be able to wield, as needed, with either the subtlety of a lancet, or the enveloping warmth of a down comforter, that was beginning to shape my ambition.

All of this had happened in just two weeks, after returning from Dallas.

Broken Whole

The Endless Night – Kicked Out of One Hotel, August 17th

These chapters might as well be subtitled "My life! My life! My life for a toothbrush!" .It is not recorded in all of human endeavor that the quest to purchase a toothbrush ever had consequences that would ultimately be as deadly as on this night of steadily unfolding disaster. But I'll get to that.

Ben's anxiety about Karma, my club idea, was a constant point of friction between us. I didn't know this at the time, but in Ben's individual meetings with Paul, our couples' therapist, Ben was breaking down, sick to his gut with fear, and Paul was telling Ben that he had to start protecting himself instead of just worrying about me. And Ben was not the only one concerned about me: Dean and I almost fell out at what I took to be his lack of support and trust in my ideas. My therapist was very worried, as were our very close friends in San Francisco. I knew all this, but none of it was enough to hold me back.

I was living in a state of fearlessness. Ben knew that I saw his anxieties as a potential drag on my progress, so he'd hold back on expressing the full extent of how he felt. There had been a few times where Ben had voiced some doubts, and I'd practically exploded, so short was my temper. One night, less than a week after the "crazy" day, I was getting ready to rush out for a meeting, and I could see the worry in Ben's face. But I mentally dismissed it, thinking it was up to him to handle his own worries. I was packing up my laptop, and I sensed Ben watching me from just a few feet away. 'Stop hovering over me!' I yelled. He blanched, and backed away. I regretted having yelled at him, but wasn't in the mood to go back on it; I was, instead, driven to get out of the door for my meeting. But as I was leaving, he started to ask me if I'd be back for dinner. In my manic state, I interpreted his question as just another attempt to control me, and I shouted at him that he should eat by himself; I didn't know when I'd be back. I was unaccountably livid with fury.

Ben was crying and shaking by now, and, as a wave of acute regret and tenderness washed away the shaking anger as if it had never been, I started towards him. To my astonishment, he backed off, visibly shaking. He was clearly terrified of me. How had it come to this, that I was capable of creating such fear in the man I loved?

Very gently, I showed him that I was no longer mad, and I slowly took him in my arms until he cried himself out. I murmured into his ear how sorry I was, and that it would never happen again. I was as appalled at my behaviour as he was.

The next day, after Ben had met with our counsellor again, Ben told me, tearfully, that he was scared of my behaviour, and observed that I, conversely, was infuriated by his anxieties. One of us should move out temporarily until we could find a better way of handling our differing perspectives on my spending and business activities. I felt secretly relieved, and told him that I agreed that it was probably the best thing for both of us. We agreed on one week apart, and that I'd move, for that duration, into the Ramada Plaza in West Hollywood. This was Wednesday night, and on Thursday, when I moved into the hotel, we agreed not to talk for a week, little knowing how soon the huge crisis, which was to begin that very night, would bring us back together. Ben and I had always considered ours a model relationship for gay couples, and had never had fears or doubts about our future together. The idea of breaking up would have seemed laughable. Yet here we were separating, even if only briefly, and all my thoughts were elsewhere, on my business ventures.

Ben spent Thursday talking to our friends, I heard later. He felt that something terrible was going to happen. I, on the other hand, went for some serious shopping in the Beverly Center. This was the day when I spent the most money, including the luggage from Prada and D&G, not to mention a complete set of DVDs of the *Star Trek* movies (which I already had at home).

Broken Whole

In the afternoon I took a break from shopping to get my hair cut by my friend, Karta, at the Beverly Peninsula. I told him that I needed an assistant, and would he be interested in working for me? (I thought it would be kind of cute when he'd be able to say, 'Hi, I'm Karta of Club Karma.') He seemed enthusiastic about the idea. (After all of this was over, Karta was added to the long list of people I had to apologize to for my behaviour.)

Outside the hotel, later, while I waited for the valet to return my car, I saw a guy getting out of a magnificent Maibach. I sauntered up to him and asked him if he owned it. He said he had a fleet of them, so I gave him my card along with the usual spiel about the club I was opening in West Hollywood. Karta and I had discussed driving together to a party in Long Beach that weekend. I asked the Maibach guy about getting a ride Saturday night, and he said he'd do it for free. This would seem to corroborate that some people, at least, took me at face value. Having said that, though, it's also possible once again that he was merely humouring me.

That night I came back to the Ramada at nine, the back of my SUV filled with shopping bags. I'd practically closed the Beverly Center, but at the last minute, I'd realized that I hadn't packed a toothbrush that morning, so I ran around the mall like a crazy person, while the shops were closing, trying to find one. I even tried Louis Vuitton, thinking they might have a luxury affair with an ebony shaft, or something equally exotic. They didn't sell toothbrushes, big surprise, but they did have a very beautiful, chic toiletries bag, which I snapped up to house the non-existent toothbrush.

It had been a long day, and I hadn't slept well for a few nights now. I had a vodka-tonic at the hotel bar, and ordered dinner. I was exhausted from frenetic activity, and the cumulative lack of sleep from almost three weeks of taking no more than two or three hours a night. I chatted for a while with a stranger I'd overheard in the Beverly Center. He had some sort of housing problem, and I'd invited him to meet me at the bar so that I could help him get everything straightened out. There wasn't a problem I believed to be too difficult for me. This was another person who took me at face value.

When I got to my room, I remembered I'd packed so quickly the night before, that I didn't have any Listerine. I also realized I needed a bottle of vodka to help slow my mind down. At this point, I needed both Xanax and vodka – taken together – to get me to sleep even for just a couple of hours each night. The drug-store was only a few blocks away, but I was too exhausted to walk, so I climbed back into my car in the parking-lot beneath the hotel.

The unfolding disaster that became the worst night of my life started off simply enough – a tussle over rules between the parking attendant, and a stubborn guest with a strong sense of justice, that is, me. I'd had a run in with this same stupid attendant, the night before, over the hotel parking card and ticket. The hotel had forgotten to give me a parking card to leave on my dash-board for the duration of my stay in the hotel. So, as I'd left the hotel the night before, all I'd had was the parking ticket which had been issued by the machine as I'd entered earlier. The parking attendant told me that I needed the dashboard card, not the parking ticket. My patience, as usual now, was so short to be non-existent, and I got very angry with him – he knew I was a guest in the hotel; couldn't he just let me out? In the end, faced with the implacability of "the rules", I conceded, and went back to the hotel to get the parking pass and ticket, muttering under my breath about insane, rule-following cretins. "The rules" would become one of themes of the dreadful night ahead.

This time, as I approached the parking attendant, my parking card on the dash-board, I knew I didn't need the orange parking ticket. But because of what had happened the night before, I was not surprised when the attendant insisted I give it to him anyway. As a hotel guest with the guest parking card, the parking ticket itself was not needed – that much I'd learned last night; I'd actually predicted to myself, as I approached him, that even though I had the parking card now, he'd still want his precious orange ticket in order to wield his tiny little piece of authority over me, hoping to bring me down to his moral stature. This too was to be one of the themes of the night. (There were many developing themes, it seemed, a sign of the vast complications that begin to adorn a manic person's life.)

I told him I'd lost the ticket, but even that wouldn't budge him. I'm not sure how he expected me to come up with a supposedly non-existent ticket (which I actually knew to be lying on my refrigerator in my suite.) Fine, I said, I'll leave my car here then, hazards on, blocking the exit barrier. I sauntered back to the hotel lobby, informed the duty manager about what was going on, and sat at my ease where I could see my car. I thought it looked fine sitting there, its front wheels turned rakishly, the slab slides of the Land Rover forming an imposing silhouette against the street lights.

The manager, who was from Eastern Europe, quickly agreed with me that I didn't need the ticket, and he called the attendant. Shortly thereafter, the manager told me it was all cleared up and I could leave without the ticket.

Now, unfortunately (this was the most destructive theme of the night), with the same very strong notion of justice that had got me into trouble in Dallas, I couldn't let the parking attendant off that easily. This was also before I'd learned another different lesson I was soon to learn: that unless you're famous, you do not get very far by messing with the system in Los Angeles. So I told the duty hotel manager that the only way my car was going to be moved from blocking the exit barrier was for the attendant to drive my car back to the valet parking area in front of the hotel lobby, and then apologize.

I'd reserved a nice suite at the hotel for a month, so I'd have expected the duty manager, seeing at least $5000 floating into the hotel from someone who didn't look like the type to mess with, to have chosen to see common business sense instead of looking at me, as he did, with a curious lack of comprehension.

Firstly, of course, I wasn't obviously famous. But I'd also failed to reckon with the manager's deep stupidity. He simply wasn't able to understand why I would make such a request. He insisted I move my car since it was blocking the exit. It was "the rules" again.

So I challenged him to call the West Hollywood Sheriff's department. About an hour later, three sheriffs arrived, listened to both sides, and, gazed rather incredulously at both of us. They were a bit surprised that I'd be prepared to push things so far, but I was also clearly winning them over to my point of view, since I was utterly calm, and the hotel staff members were all so excitable. ('Foreigners!' I thought to myself, thinking of old British movies.)

While waiting for the sheriffs to arrive, I'd cancelled my reservation at the Ramada, and had tried to book a room elsewhere. But even more celebrities were arriving in LA for some very important sort of show ("The Enormities"?), so nothing was available. Although, even then, of course, if I'd been famous, I could have still probably got a room at the Peninsula in Beverly Hills, especially if the magnitude of my celebrity outranked that of, say, a minor soap star from the Valley.

After much bargaining, I refused to budge my position, and the evening ended with no apology from the attendant, a loss of $5000 to the hotel, and the sheriffs and I becoming buddies. They packed all my stuff, and helped me load it into my car, which they'd themselves moved from the exit barrier to the valet parking spot outside the lobby. I said my final goodbye forever to the Ramada West Hollywood, and was let out by the thoroughly disgruntled attendant.

The Endless Night – Kicked Out of a Second Hotel, August 18th

When I left the Ramada, I called several hotels downtown, and found that none of them had rooms. Meanwhile, in the back of my mind, running at full pitch again, a new plan had been percolating. I was still operating under the thesis that I'd become a powerful, multidimensional person in a matter of days, after half a life of chronic depression. It was a massive transformation of a type probably never recorded before, I believed. The week in Dallas; the day I conceived my customer-service idea and then almost went crazy trying to get to Ben; my certainty of soon opening a club in West Hollywood; and even tonight's events at the Ramada in West Hollywood: all of these loomed as signposts along a trajectory of explosive growth. Outlandish as the ideas seem, I sincerely believed that my story would be told in scientific journals, and that news and television outlets would be clamouring for my attention.

I suddenly thought: why do I need to stay in Los Angeles right now? I was beginning to find it toxic. I have many friends in San Francisco, I thought. I'll just spend the night in Los Angeles and then fly to San Francisco for a few weeks, all thoughts of the "trial" one-week separation from Ben forgotten. I called the W in San Francisco, and booked a corner suite for a month. I imagined that I would immediately try to find the best available writer to work on my book as a ghost.

Meanwhile, there was still the issue of finding a hotel for the night, and this led to what would be another manic, obsessive quest like those that had bedeviled me in Dallas. Somebody had told me to try the W Hotel, downtown on 3rd Street, so, enormously tired, I got on the freeway heading downtown, and called directory enquiries to get their number. But the W wasn't listed, and I therefore assumed the hotel was brand new. I'd been given the address, so, once I was off the freeway, I tried to program it into my car's navigation system. To my astonishment, it maintained the address didn't exist. I set off to try to find it by driving. However the streets in downtown Los Angeles are very hard to navigate, since most streets are one-way, there are two freeways cutting through, and some of the streets which appear a solid part of earth when you're driving them are actually revealed to be elevated. I kept circling the general area where I knew Third Street must begin, but could never quite get to the block where I was sure the W Hotel must exist. I pulled over a couple of times to ask people, and got frustrated when they couldn't seem to understand that a hotel could be called W. In my intense fatigue, I was past caring about the rules of the road; it was late at night, so I gently rolled through multiple-red lights and performed illegal u-turns until I finally came upon a stub of Third Street that dead-ended just before the freeway. There was clearly no hotel. Even then the mania-fueled determination that there was no such thing as insolvable conundrum forced me to search for other solutions. I temporarily parked my car with the valet at the nearby Omni Hotel, and hailed a cab. Why I believed a rude, squalid looking cabbie could find a hotel called W (no hotel called W, he muttered) better than I could is not immediately obvious to me now. The downtown W simply didn't exist. It had taken me two hours of increasing frustration to come to this conclusion, when it should have been immediately obvious after directory enquires had no listing. Yet the hotel had to exist, I'd told myself, and I would find it, no matter how difficult they made it to find.

But now, having finally accepted the inevitable conclusion, feeling irate and completely shredded – almost in panic at the extent of my fatigue, I returned to the Omni, and asked them if they had any rooms. I honestly didn't know what I would do if they didn't have a room.

'Please tell me you have a room.'

I managed a grin, despite everything. At the front-desk was a kindly-looking, middle-aged, chicly dressed

African-American. She smiled back, after a quick check of her system.

'You're in luck, we have one room left!'

With immense relief, I pulled out my credit card holder, gave her my credit card, and then saw, to my absolute horror, that my driver's license – which, by now, I'd recovered from the bank – was missing: I'd lost it yet again, this time after setting up my fifth charge account of the days at Louis Vuitton, in the Beverly Center, in order to buy the toiletries back in place of the toothbrush they didn't sell.

'I don't have my license,' I stammered. I looked through all my pockets. 'Is that a problem?' I asked her.

She grimaced apologetically. 'I'm afraid so, Mr. Adams.'

I looked at her with desperation. 'Can you please make an exception? I'm completely exhausted.'

When it was obvious that she couldn't be moved, I abruptly collapsed to the floor, dramatically, physically and emotionally shattered, weeping. This was much to my own surprise, as well as much to the alarm of the receptionist. I'd not cried like this in twenty years. In fact, in twenty years, I'd barely shed any tears at all. This was the night that would teach me how to cry again.

At first the receptionist took pity on me. She led me to a sofa, and allowed me time to pull myself together. But eventually she called three security guards, who approached me in the middle of the lobby, as I lay on the sofa.

'We're going to have to ask you to leave, sir.'

I looked at them incredulously.

'Let me just call another hotel, maybe they'll take me in.'

The head security guard was a spindly man with a scrawny beard looking not unlike a cross-breed between Jesus and a rodent. He shook his head. 'I'm sorry, sir.' He gestured at the exit.

I'd completely recovered my composure by now, and my feistiness.

'I'm not moving,' I said.

Now it was their turn to stare incredulously.

'If you want me to leave, you're going to have to carry me out.'

They looked at each other then moved towards me, pulling me up, one guard carrying my legs, the other two, an arm each. I genuinely thought it was quite hilarious: they seemed to think they were winning a big victory over me, and that I was surrendering my dignity, whereas, in my view, they were, as is the norm for Los Angeles, more concerned about appearances – in this case their nice hotel lobby – than about having the common human decency to help a person in need. As at the Ramada, I was sure I was in the right. They thought they'd made me look ridiculous, while, inside, I was laughing at them for their petty victories: not one shred of my dignity or sense of self was pricked.

The situation, however, was devolving eerily into what had happened earlier at the Ramada. The behaviour of the security guards was mostly influenced by the head guard, who I'd started calling Weasel-Face, in my mind. I could sense in him the need to repudiate his inner feelings of powerlessness; the same feelings that had motivated the parking guy at the Ramada. He was going to satisfy this need whatever it took, especially now that he'd attempted to humiliate me and had utterly failed.

Once I was outside, in the courtyard of the hotel, I immediately realized that because of my breakdown at the front desk I'd left my credit-card holder with them. Defying any rational explanation, Weasel-Face would neither let me enter the hotel to retrieve my credit cards nor bring them out to me. I then realized that, of course, the valet had the keys to my car, which was parked in the hotel courtyard, just a few feet from where I was sitting on the curb. The idiocy of the situation became complete when Weasel-Face also refused to let the valet give me back my keys.

His two associates seemed like reasonable men, but wouldn't override Weasel; and the valet was secure behind a window, and wouldn't follow any instructions except those given by Weasel. And of course I couldn't get into the hotel to reason with the woman at the reception desk about my credit cards. The hotel was clearly in the wrong; they had no right to deprive me of my belongings. But no amount of reasoning or negotiation could produce from them a valid reason for their behaviour. I asked them to call the hotel manager; they refused. I met with the same blank refusal when I asked them to summon the police. (Of course, how could they do either of these two things? It would result in my belongings being returned to me, they would be proven to have been in the wrong, and they would have lost their supposed moral victory.)

Weasel's ostensible, stated reason for denying me my belongings was that I appeared to be high. I could understand why they might think so; my eyes must have been blazing with manic intensity, not to mention red-rimmed with overwhelming fatigue. Nonetheless, I was completely eloquent and cogent in my arguments, and perfectly capable of driving. And in any case, none of that mattered: the plain facts were that even if I was high they couldn't appropriate my property. Moreover, if they really believed I was high, and that my driving would endanger others, surely they'd call the police.

Time passed. My new cell-phone – bought for a second time now after I'd tossed the first one into a parking lot on my mad trek across Hollywood – was somewhere in my car, so I couldn't call the police myself. (Was it really only a week since I'd bought it the first time on the day where I went unhinged?) I no longer had any idea what time it was, except that it was late - too late for any foot or street traffic, let alone a taxi. My blood began to boil: I was going to make them call the police. I returned to the hotel courtyard, and started shouting very loudly. I knew that the last thing a hotel like this wanted was for paying guests to witness any part of this scene. So I yelled and shouted, long enough for the security guards to be forced to try to stop me. I promised to stop if they would call the police, and they agreed. But I could see in their eyes that it was very doubtful they'd follow through on their promise. And sure enough, the police never came.

I upped the ante, pretending to have a heart attack on the sidewalk outside of the hotel. I really threw my heart into it, so to speak, ending the performance by lying motionless for over a minute. For the first time in my life, I gave a completely authentic acting performance, something I'd never achieved in any of my acting classes. They didn't buy it. Ironic, I thought, that in this town famous for acting, I should give my best ever performance to a disinterested party of three.

I tried a couple of other tricks: I lay for a while in the centre of the road. It was surprisingly comfortable, and I even contemplated the idea of falling asleep. But apart from being restful, it was not moving me towards my goal of getting the police involved, since there was no traffic. Then I walked down the street, peering into office-building lobbies to see if I could find a security guard whom I could persuade to call the police. I did persuade one guard to unlock his doors and talk to me. I explained to him that the hotel down the street was keeping my car keys and my credit cards; could he call the police for me? He just looked at me uncertainly, and then made as if to close the door. I stopped him and ask what I would have to do to get him to call the police. He locked the door on me; so I ran across the street and calculatedly kicked the plastic sheeting covering a large poster on the side of a bus shelter repeatedly, as hard as I could. I watched him go back to his desk. He did nothing.

The situation was Kafkaesque. Here I was, in my own city, my boyfriend presumably asleep in my bed (more likely lying awake worrying about me), my car right in front of me, yet no means of finding shelter for the night. And since I was more tired than I'd ever been in my life, shelter was all that I craved. The only line I wouldn't cross was that I wouldn't pull Ben into the situation. And in any case, even if I had wanted to involve Ben, I had neither my cell-phone, nor the energy to trudge the streets in search of a pay-phone, even if there was a single working pay-phone in downtown Los Angeles, which I doubted.

One final resort came to me as I suddenly remembered, belatedly, that I'd left the car unlocked when I'd dropped it at the valet. My money clip – bought at Vuitton just today, or rather yesterday, now hours and hours ago – was in the car, holding hundreds of dollars. I could load my luggage onto one of the hotel luggage carts, along with the many bags of shopping I'd acquired earlier in the day, push the luggage cart to the curb, and wait until dawn when, presumably, taxi cabs would appear. It was far from an ideal solution, but it appealed to me because it would at least foil Weasel.

Because, in the past, I'd never considered myself physically courageous, the current situation - as I knew it would unfold - showed me more than anything else how much I'd changed recently. I knew this final confrontation would end in a fist-fight, and I relished the idea. I knew exactly what was going to happen. I pushed the luggage trolley towards the car; the three security guards inserted themselves, inevitably, between trolley and car, but I kept on moving. When the trolley hit them, they launched at me. Unlike during all my fist-fights at high-school, my physical coordination did not desert me. I had the intense satisfaction of seeing my large fist land squarely on Weasel's jaw. But I was outnumbered; I was also incredibly exhausted; more important, one of them was tall, young and strong. I was soon immobilized face down, and I stopped resisting. But Weasel hadn't had enough: for a couple of minutes he stood on the nape of my neck and continued to punch me. In other words, on Omni Hotel property, where my possessions had been effectively stolen from me by Omni staff, one of their employees assaulted me with the intent of harming me while I was restrained by two others. As I lay there, face-down, I now knew, finally, where the most immediate source of money was going to come from: this was a law-suit in waiting.

He left his foot there, pushing my face into the ground, until the LAPD finally arrived. As a formality, since the hotel had called them, I was arrested, cuffed, and put into the back of the cruiser, while the police talked to the security guards. I watched closely, and could see the looks of perplexity on the faces of the two policemen. I imagined the security guards were having a hard time explaining why they'd kept me from my property.

My sense of the situation was confirmed once the police interviewed me. We chatted on the way over to the station. Even in this extremity of fatigue, I could still muster an engaging manner, and seemingly win people over to my side. And they'd been kind enough to retrieve my cell-phone from my car before we'd left the hotel.

It was ironic – given how I'd driven earlier in the evening on the way to the hotel – that they politely asked me if I minded if they ran a few red lights. They agreed that the security guards had behaved irrationally, but were still obliged to take me into the station. They said I'd be in and out in half an hour. In fact, I was about to enter the real part of the nightmare.

Broken Whole

The Endless Night – LAPD Lockup, August 18th

Once inside the jail, still cuffed, I was placed in a holding cell, and divested of all my personal belongings, except my commitment ring, which I refused to give up. The two cops who had arrested me were kind, but the paperwork seemed endless. Finally, I was led out to a booking room, containing some seats, and a window at which a different pair of cops were completing the paperwork for the seedy looking guy they'd arrested. Never having had any contact with the criminal justice system apart from what I'd seen on television and in movies (many of them, of course, involving the LAPD), it felt extremely odd to be about to participate in the ritual I was witnessing, which indeed looked familiar from TV. I was rather dazed. There seemed to be interminable complications to the process, with all the cops looking bored and restless.

As I sat waiting on the bench, one of the other cops, a beefy, spunky looking lesbian, unknowingly brushed her boot back and forth over the metal leg of her stool. She was completely unconscious of what she was doing, but in my loneliness, the soft repetitive thud of her boot against the chair sounded to me like the heartbeat of humanity, and gave me hope. I even told her so, not that there was a hope she'd understand what I meant. Even now, my desire to connect was undiminished.

Before I was processed, I was allowed to make a phone call. The rules for using the phone were very complicated. I racked my brain for any number that wasn't Ben's. I still hoped to keep him out of this (his previous bipolar boyfriend had been jailed twice). But I finally realized tearfully there was no choice; Ben was the only person who could help me. I called him, and told him what had happened. Ben is somebody prone to emotional reactions, and occasional panic, and I was surprised by how calm he sounded. This was to be the only connection I was allowed to make to anybody I knew for another twenty-four hours.

Eventually it was my turn to be processed, and the paperwork was completed. I was photographed and fingerprinted, and photographs were taken of the bruises caused by the fight. I was, by this time, so deeply fatigued that I could barely move. They gave me a piece of paper on which I managed to scrawl a semblance of my signature, and handed me a pink copy, but since I was too tired even to accept the paper in my hand, they stuffed it into one of my pockets. They took the handcuffs off me, and directed me towards what looked like an exit, where they said I'd be given my cell-phone. I shuffled over there, all but dead on my feet.

The new room I'd been led into – more of a tiny corridor than a room – turned out to be locked at both ends, with an open grille looking back into the booking room where I'd just been photographed. I was not given my cell-phone. Although I felt as if I'd been tricked, I sat patiently for what seemed like an hour. Finally, I spoke to the officer nearest the grille.

'I thought I was going to get my cell-phone?' My voice sounded rather pathetic, I thought.

He mumbled something about needing the pink ticket, and I scrambled through my jeans and found it, and pushed it out through the bars.

'Nobody told me I had to do anything with it,' I complained.

This was when I realized that something was very wrong. The officer practically snarled at me. 'Next time you should listen?'

I was a man who'd been pushed to the edge, as if I'd been in a war zone; I started to cry. It alarmed me how easily I could cry all of a sudden, and, as I concluded days later, there is nothing more likely to aggravate an LAPD officer than a man crying.

'Can't you understand how tired I am? I'm sorry I didn't hear what you said,' I managed to get out.

What happened next is a bit of a blur, but I do know that they cleared out, not just a jail cell, but an entire jail block. They cuffed me to lead me to one of the freed up cells, which had presumably been holding several men just minutes earlier, took my handcuffs off again, and locked the door behind me. I still don't understand why they thought I was so dangerous.

I was still (though I didn't recognize it) in the grip of the manic phase of my first bipolar swing. I'd been in a increasingly manic state since San Diego, and each day, I'd probably experienced hundreds of times more thoughts than I was used to experiencing. It was now mid-day Friday, and I hadn't been to bed since Wednesday night. For several days previously, I'd had not much more than a couple of hours sleep each night, and each one of those days had been filled with feverish intellectual and physical activity. I'd spent a good portion of Thursday shopping (which is, admittedly, not that intellectual but nonetheless exhausting), and that night there had been the incident at the Ramada, and then the long affair at the Omni Hotel, which had culminated in the fight that had got me arrested. At the moment they cleared out the cell block and locked me up again, I'd been awake about thirty hours, during which time I'd been through the most intense experiences of my life. Because of the rapidity of my thought processes, every minute spent in that cell seemed like an eternity.

My heart was racing. It was hot, and I took off my shirt and doused my body with water. Every now and then I'd hear the clinking of keys as a jailer approached, and my heart would leap, and then sink again as the sound dwindled. I wept and felt intolerably alone in the hot cell where nobody could hear me when I yelled, which I did frequently. I couldn't understand why I hadn't been released. I literally thought I was going to die in that cell.

Not knowing police procedures, and still clinging to the promise made by the arresting cops that I'd be out quickly, I couldn't comprehend why Ben wasn't here to bail me out. After all, it all looked so easy – and relatively inconsequential – on *Beverly Hills 90210* when somebody got bailed out. Indeed scenes like that were often used for comedy. There was nothing in the least bit comedic about it for me, and I'm ashamed to say I felt some very bitter thoughts about Ben's seeming absence.

The phone in the cell didn't work according to the same system as the one I'd used earlier to call Ben. A passing, obviously psychopathic cop told me I hadn't listened to them, because the code to use the phone, although different from the other phone code, had been explained to me. I begged him to explain it to me, but didn't have an ounce of anything but contempt for what he saw as my weakness.

I did eventually learn the supposedly correct code, but also learned it could not be used to call cell-phones. There wasn't a single land-line in my memory. Nonetheless, although I was so tired I had to hold myself up by leaning against the phone, I stood at the phone many long minutes, randomly dialing numbers in the hope of reaching somebody, anybody who could help me, such was my loneliness and desperation. All I got was the busy signal. I don't think that phone worked at all.

Despite my fatigue, my mind was still running so hot that I felt I'd been eight hours in that cell, when in fact it may well have been as few as two. I felt that, for no reason I could understand, I'd been locked up, and the key thrown away.

I wept many times, groaned and roared with frustration, rattled the bars, trying to make a ruckus. Once, a cleaning woman went past, and I again faked having a heart attack. I swear she didn't miss a single mote of dust. Later, when a female cop passed, I managed to persuade her I was close to having a heart attack, which, after all the fake ones, this time seemed to me to be true. She brought back the psychopathic cop who'd poured scorn on me earlier. He looked at me in disgust. 'Be a man', he said, and walked away.

When my medical condition was finally taken seriously, I was cuffed again, this time with the cuffs behind my back. They were cruelly tight for my large wrists. I was led back to the holding cell next to the booking room; then taken into a medical room to see two nurses who took my blood pressure. In the cell, before they'd come for me, I'd deliberately excited myself internally in the hope of increasing it, so I was hoping that it was dangerously high.

But the nurses gave me no information; nor did they prescribe any type of medication. I was moved back to my original holding cell, in the same cuffed posture. This cell was at least an improvement over the distant cell-room I'd just come from, and I felt, since it was next to the processing room, that it was likely to be closer to where Ben was. It was furnished only with a wooden bench. I was completely depleted of all strength, barely able to walk. The only way I could find rest was to lower myself carefully backwards onto the bench. But in that position, the cuffs bit into my lower back, leaving bruises and pain that lasted for weeks. The cuffs were so tight that my hands were turning blue. The irony would not have been lost on me – had I had the energy to think of it – that it had been painful decades of hatred of my physical being, precipitated by my dad's comment on my skinny wrists, that had contributed to depression, and had possibly led directly to this moment where I thought I was in danger of dying because my wrists were too large for the hand-cuffs.

I tried, really tried, to be patient, but hours seemed to pass. They told me that Ben was just next door, and, not knowing the layout of the place, I thought he was maybe just through the far door that the cops used to exit the booking room. Each time that door opened, I'd yell Ben's name through the grille of the holding cell's door, hoping he'd hear me.

From time to time, I'd sink to the floor and weep again, feeling hopeless and wretched. I had no idea how things had come to this, nor what to do about it, nor how it would end, if ever. I thought I might not make it. It seemed endless. I slammed my cuffs against the grille, careless that I might further damage my wrists and back, trying to wear out the patience of the cops in the booking room. My heart-rate began to accelerate again, and once more I felt in fear of having a heart attack, with the cuffs cutting off my circulation. I demanded medical attention, and they kept saying I'd seen the doctor thirty minutes ago, which, by then, was clearly a lie. I faked another Oscar-worthy heart attack, my third of the evening, which was ignored as the first two had been. I began to feel they wanted me to either die, or commit suicide: anything to release them from responsibility over me.

    I was in a dangerous condition of desperation, prepared to do almost anything to get out of that cell. When an officer temporarily opened the door to my cell, I thrust my foot through the opening to prevent him from closing it. Everybody tensed up. I knew I was endangering myself, but I had to get out of there, and get medical attention, or reach Ben. I asked them if I could see my doctor, Ben (who holds an M.D.). I watched with all my concentration to see if any of the cops were going for their guns, or night-sticks. The stand-off didn't last long: I didn't have the strength to hold the door open, and they were able to push my foot back inside. But the incident must have impressed upon them that I clearly believed I was medically at risk; so they offered me the opportunity of attention from the same nurses I'd seen earlier. I refused, saying I'd only see my own doctor (that is, my boyfriend). Naively, I thought they'd have no choice but to let me see Ben. But that just wasn't going to fly. Apparently the nurses then went to talk to Ben.

    I wanted desperately to reach Ben, to let him know I was nearby, and that I knew he was near me. I struck up a conversation with a Hispanic cop, and, despite my intense fatigue, my mind was now working again at a furious pitch, and my eyes must have burned. I exerted every ounce of my ingenuity and strength, mustering a fierce, almost daemonic trance, which I exerted on this poor, not overly bright cop. He didn't stand a chance. By constant intellectual argument, and manic intensity, I had him convinced that I was capable of seeing his soul. I made him believe that he, alone of all the cops in the facility, had a shred of a soul left, and that he could rescue that soul from destruction. There was not an argument that he could muster that I couldn't instantly contradict with a telling blow.

Finally, once I had him in my hand, I let slip my commitment-ceremony-ring so that it fell into his side of the room. I told him that he could save his soul from destruction by simply picking up my ring, stepping next door, and giving it to Ben.

But that would be breaking the rules, he said.

I knew that I could be really hurting this man; and he knew it too. He seemed to be good-hearted – indeed the only such cop I came into contact with that night. I didn't want to hurt him, but I felt an inconceivable urgency to get out of the cell, whatever it took. The poor man kept gripping his head, saying, 'Oh man, you're messing with my head.' Other people, mostly janitorial staff members, were also watching, transfixed by the scene. I'd never, at any time in my life, been more focused and present than I was right then, intent on forcing this man to my will, even from my position of apparent helplessness.

I pulled his partner into the conversation, a German-American blond guy, surnamed Weh, primed with the bravado and cruelty that was written on his features. He tried to goad me, and humiliate me, but I wouldn't be overridden. I told him that I could see right into his head.

'What do you see,' he asked.

'Nothing,' I replied. 'You have no soul.'

After more exchanges like this, he tried to laugh me off, but wouldn't meet my eyes.

'Do you know any German?' I asked him.

'No,' he said.

'Do you know what your surname means?'

'No.'

'The word *weh*, means *empty*.' (It doesn't.)

A certain chill entered their eyes. My eyes and my relentless argument tore into them, for I was desperate. In the end, almost inconceivably, I had both of them convinced that I was the Anti-Christ, and that they had two choices: one was to hand the ring to Ben; the other was to suffer the extinguishing of their souls by placing it on my finger. I was in the grip of manic brilliance: these two cops were so scared that neither of them would put the ring on my finger

They were saved from eternal damnation when, eventually, the sergeant, realizing how dangerous my words were, reassigned the two cops.

My heart was racing again, and I was increasingly desperate. I knew I needed medical attention, or else I'd probably have a heart attack or a brain aneurysm, and there was only one trick left to pull. I announced at the top of my voice, that at the count of ten I would commit suicide. I counted down very loudly, increasingly slowly. At the count of 'one', I sought for a way to make it seem like I could do it. But I could find no way of making it look plausible. I was too weak to climb up onto anything to act as if I was going to plunge to the ground head first, and, besides, with my hands shackled behind my back, there was no way I could even climb. I collapsed on the floor and wept more bitterly than ever.

For the first time, the sergeant voluntarily spoke to me through the grille in the door. It seemed impossible, but suddenly I was about to be released, but to a medical facility, not to my partner and freedom. They'd evidently believed I was suicidal; my ploy had worked in so far as it did lead to my getting out of jail. However it had ended, wholly unexpectedly, with my being strapped into a gurney. As I was led by kindly medical orderlies to the ambulance, I realized it was a beautiful late summer evening, almost twenty-four hours after the first incident of the evening, at the Ramada. I was endlessly thankful that Ben was not there to witness me tied to a gurney as if I was a crazy person. It was completely beyond my comprehension, however, that I had only been in jail for eight hours: it had felt like more than twenty-four.

I suddenly remembered, with panic, my commitment ring, still on the floor of the processing room! But somebody else had had the same thought. The Hispanic cop who'd seemed the only cop to show me any heart – the same cop whose head I'd messed with – came up to the gurney, and, without saying anything or making eye-contact, he slipped my ring into the pocket of my jeans.

I whispered to him urgently, 'Find a new partner!'

The Endless Night – in the Psychiatric System, August 18th to 21st

If anybody had ever asked me, I'd have said that the chances of me ever ending up in a mental hospital were zero. Sure, I felt, in some ways, that I understood insanity. As a very introspective person, I'd spent enough time in my head that I felt I could perceive the fine line between sanity and madness. And, on two occasions, in my adult life, I'd felt on the edge of losing myself in a whirlpool of depression. On the day when I'd almost gone crazy trying to make the couples' counselling meeting with Ben, I'd felt perilously close to insanity. But looking back, I'm no longer sure that I was truly at risk. If there is one claim I feel I can honestly make about myself, it's that I understand myself more than the average person. I had enough smarts to get me through that crisis; and I had too strong a pride to ever give in completely to depression, even if it meant I had to fight it for the rest of my life.

Yet after being released from those horrible eight hours in jail, I spent three days locked away in the psychiatric system. I wasn't, in fact, dangerous to myself or to anybody else, nor was I so ill in the head that I required full-time treatment. I was locked up because it had appeared that I was suicidal when I was in jail. I'd pretended to be suicidal in order to get medical treatment, and, hopefully, so that the LAPD would let me see Ben. It had never occurred to me that I might get locked up in a mental hospital as a result.

The night had been the longest of my life and I was grateful it was over. But it had scared me that the ER team taking me from the jail thought it was necessary to strap me to a gurney, immobilizing my arms and legs. And I'd been worried that Ben would see me like this, and it would fuel his worry.

My worry proved unnecessary. The two medics were kind and patient with me, and told me I wasn't going to see my family today; I had to go for an evaluation first at the psychiatric ER.

On the way to the ER, I talked with the female medic. I still hadn't slept in two days, and was still manic; but I was concerned, above all else, that people didn't think I was anything other than normal. I told her all of the theories I was coming up with to explain what had happened to me; I told her about my boyfriend and how he and all my friends had been needlessly worried about me. And she listened. She was bipolar herself, and, as I later realized, she went along with my ideas, as she was trained to do. One thing I learned through this whole period was that I wasn't very good at recognizing when I was being humoured.

At the ER, I was held for a long time, still strapped in the gurney, outside the ward, so that the staff could perform the intake functions. The idea of being restrained like this was completely at odds with my world view. I was worried at the noise coming from the ER: shouting and anger. I was having an extreme disconnect. How could I be a part of this? I was eventually given a hospital gown, my restraints were removed, and I walked into the ER ward. The doors were locked behind me. In the ward, the few patients who were awake looked over at me with expressionless faces.

I was practically dead on my feet with fatigue, the ward was freezing, and the television blared. I think it was the television that disturbed me the most: I hated television with a passion, and would do virtually anything to avoid having to listen to its commercial blather; and now it looked as if I might have to suffer through it for many hours.

Even though I didn't want to be near the other patients, I found an empty bed, and hid myself under the thin blanket. But sleep wouldn't come.

They gave me food, but I couldn't stomach it, despite my not having eaten in almost twenty-four hours: cold, plastic pasta and cardboard vegetables.

I hadn't showered in two days, and during that time I'd been beaten up, and then jailed: I wanted badly to take a shower, despite how chilly the room was. But they had a push-button shower: each cycle would last no more than twenty seconds, not long enough for it to even get lukewarm, even if you repeated the process several times in a row.

The poverty of the service, and the obvious lack of empathy exhibited in its design made me realize how powerless the seriously mentally ill are (not that I yet considered myself amongst them.) Nobody cared to think that these people were human beings, in need of the same basics as anybody else: comfort, warmth, decent food, and an opportunity for dignity.

I asked for medication so that I could sleep, but I was told they couldn't give me anything until the psychologist arrived.

To pass the time, I talked with Tamika, the orderly watching over the ward. She was kind, if a little stern. Every time I thought of what I'd been through, and, most especially, the grief I'd caused for my friends, I'd cry, and Tamika would chide me for not being manly. I didn't take it personally. Crying was such a relief. I took it as a new found strength that I could finally cry so easily after all these years. She did, however, show me the DSM-IV criteria for a manic episode, something that gave me a lot to think about.

I have a mortal fear of being unoccupied, and since I had nothing to read, I asked for paper and pen. Even that had to be negotiated, since it was against the precious rules. I suppose I might have stabbed myself in the throat with a ball-point pen. However, they relented, and I began to write. My mind, still completely unrested after two nights, was overflowing with ideas and conclusions both about what had happened to me, and about my place in the universe.

To start off with, there were things I needed to say to friends and family. I wrote:

> *The idea has started to form in my mind that maybe my friends have been partially correct. Over the past few weeks (and bear in mind I've not had a*

trace of depression now in three months after battling it for most of my adult life), I've already admitted to one day's dalliance with insanity. Now, I'm ready to admit that I did also have moments or hours of partial mania. Bear in mind that even full blown manic depression is not necessarily a severe mental illness. Its relationship to bipolar disorder (a serious illness) is the same as major depression is to moderate depression (what I've experienced for a decade and a half)[3]. I now admit that at times I've certainly possessed seven of the eleven symptoms of mania.

Another thing in my favour: the poles through which I've swung have been between excessively high, and just plain old high; rather than between excessively high and a bad crash.

However, I question whether or not borderline mania is just a different (perhaps better?) method of coping with the world around us. After all, if the universe was created as a bipolar singularity – an infinitely tiny point at one moment, the next spreading into infinity – and we're on the path to the void, couldn't you say that a happy medium between mania and normality is indeed the most rational response to the current state of the universe?

And I wrote poems and essays: conclusions about my behaviour and my life going forward. One of them was called: *Letting Go.*

I'd begun to believe my own witchcraft – that the right combination of fearlessness, looks, charms, money and intellect could let you achieve almost

---

[3] I was wrong here: manic depression is just another name for bipolar disorder.

anything. In fact, almost everywhere except Los Angeles, you'd almost be correct. Moreover, anywhere else you'd probably not need all of them.

Even outside Los Angeles, there are certain natural limits to these lesser powers, including fame. One of those limits is time. Those powers can probably get you anything you want – eventually – but maybe not soon enough. Another is stupidity, which is of key importance. Never underestimate the power of a deeply stupid person to misunderstand when they should be scratching your back while you're scratching theirs.

A final, very important limiting factor is that people hate to feel that their powers, however petty, cannot affect you, so they will stick to "not breaking the rules" no matter how obvious it is that only a foolish man clings to rules even when they're clearly to his disadvantage.

I saw this in a very minor way, for instance, combined with the effects of celebrity, at the Peninsula, Beverly Hills, a very famous luxury hotel, where I'd stopped off to visit my charming friend Karta, who's a true artist and gentleman in the Salon there. While waiting to ask the concierge a question, an older, conservatively dressed but clearly wealthy couple asked about outdoor Italian dining in the area. Naively convinced, still, that charm could work anywhere, I told them about Bienvenuto in West Hollywood, a beautiful place with a double deck. Their eyes swivelled to me, and looked me up and down. I watched an internal sniff being displayed on their bovine features, and without even acknowledging me, they returned to talk with the concierge. No karma, I thought to myself, smiling.

Broken Whole

Yet even in Los Angeles, the well-grounded can flourish; witness all of my friends, and other people I met that same day at the Peninsula Hotel. But even groundedness cannot help people unfortunate enough to get involved with "the system." For if you're like me, and you encounter the system, and you have a strong drive to right wrong, you may get deeply fucked. This means, for me personally, because of my nature, and because of the nature of Los Angeles, I have to start letting things go. I can't right every wrong here.

Take my encounter with the Ramada Hotel, the Omni Hotel downtown, and my subsequent arrest by the LAPD. From my point of view, I was right all along the way. But what was the cost to my friends and family? Too heavy.

I was feeling a bitter hatred for the LAPD, an institution I now thought of as deeply broken. I saw a parallel to my realization that my new laptop had become too complex to function effectively. Similarly, I thought, the LAPD was too bloated to do its job with any humanity. Complexity could not coexist with simplicity.

To try to encapsulate what I was feeling, I wrote another poem. It was called *broken whole (a theory of everything)*, and postulated that nothing could be simultaneously complex and whole, except a grounded human being, or the singularity that began the universe.

Since nothing was perfect since the universe began, the singularity proceeds ineluctably to chaos then void.

Pebbles make tiny splashes in the ocean, tsunamis ashore. Just so, infinitesimal flaws in the early (not initial since that was whole) moments of time, led to the Sun, and the Milky Way; all fading now.

This illustrates connectedness near and far, integration too. Everything is seemingly random, yet becomes fatefully causal.

We see this all the time: a kindly small-town sheriff bloats into the broken LAPD (which tried and failed to delete my soul tonight with all their power in their downtown citadel.)

Some might call it whole, yet the LAPD cannot be fixed: can it be unbroken? Remember, chaos cloaked the initial singularity (and we all know where that went).

So can integral complexity exist? It certainly did once: in the singularity, which, by the way, had two poles: universe and void. In its way, it was like The One, a grounded human being: the most (the only?) perfect creation between the singularity and chaos.

Later, I'd write:

I may have cried, many times, but they never broke me. The beautiful J Lindberg shirt I'm wearing – ripped during the mêlée at the Omni – will always remain precious to me: my badge of honor that I stood up to the LAPD, the most fearsome police force in the world.

I'd been allowed to talk to Ben on the phone, and had asked him to bring warm clothes, protein bars, a toothbrush and toothpaste, and some books and magazines. Finally, I was allowed to see Ben and Dean. My heart broke as the orderly opened the door to the ward and I saw the look of haunted anxiety on Ben's face. He was deathly pale. We both broke down, but Ben wasn't allowed in the room, and I wasn't allowed out, so we had only a minute or two to hug each other and talk. I was very urgent about wanting out. At this point I didn't realize that the psychiatric ER was not my last port of call in the system.

I cried when I hugged Dean too: I felt awful about what he'd gone through as my closest friend. Dean had been intimately involved with both of us, together and individually, through the long build up of my manic phase. Neither of us could have got through this period without Dean's strength, intellect, care and affection. Even on the day he visited me, Dean was pulling strings behind the scenes to get me released to a non-ER facility. I'd asked them to make sure I got a private room, since I knew I wouldn't be able to sleep if there was somebody else in my room.

Things went easier for me after they left. The television was switched off, and I had food, and something to read. Yet, for the first time in my life, I couldn't seem to focus on a book. My mind was still sparkling with ideas and concepts, and I'd lose track of the book within the first paragraph.

So I started watching the other patients. Oddly enough, they didn't seem terribly strange. Two of them were clearly very intelligent, and played cards together. I felt a surprising kinship with each of them. The young man would blaze into fury if his wishes weren't immediately met: a reminder of my own towering impatience with just about every obstacle in the previous few weeks. And the girl had an exquisite modulation to every single word she uttered, as if trying to imbue everything with the perfect pitch required to either make her point, or be understood. I recognized that as being similar to the way I'd been interacting with strangers over the last few weeks: how I'd felt an almost mystical sense that I could predict and therefore control to my own ends the entire course of a conversation.

That evening – Friday night – I was moved to a locked inpatient psychiatric ward in Torrance. I was sure it would be for one night only. I'd clearly won over the staff of the ER, and surely they'd tell the doctors that I wasn't crazy, or a risk to myself. I was horrified, when I arrived, though, to find that I didn't have a room to myself after all. In fact, I was to share it with a guy who looked like a street-person, who acted as if he was perpetually drunk, and who grumbled and groaned, speaking to himself, for as long as I could bear to be in the same room as him.

My fears about what I'd find inside the ward had been almost immediately confirmed: the patients seemed comically stereotypical, as if they'd been cast as crazy people on a TV movie of the week. There was *the preacher*, who was always accompanied by his bible when he gave his stern lectures. There was a guy who hectored the staff every half an hour in a stentorian roar, 'Smoke time, smoke time?' There was the guy who fondled the other patients. He ran his hand over my backside when I was standing in line, that night, waiting to get my sleeping medication, and I punched him in the arm. It never even occurred to me until after I'd done it that perhaps it could get me into trouble. But the staff members were used both to him and the reactions he provoked, and blithely admonished him.

I knew I didn't belong there. The staff knew I didn't belong there, or so it seemed to me. But I never felt that I was above the other patients. I knew that if I allowed myself to feel empathy for them, I could get sucked in, so I kept my distance. I greatly admired the patience of the staff members: they treated each patient as an individual, not as a child.

Sleep still didn't come to me, even though by now, I'd been given a sedative, and hadn't slept in three nights. I got to talking with an intelligent, friendly young orderly who was guarding the entrance to the women's quarters. He happened to share my interest in cosmology, so I read him a short poetic essay I'd written earlier that night, *Get Integrated (a guide to the soul)*. It was a stretch of an analogy about superstring theory and the evolution of an enlightened soul[4]. (Michio Kaku was speaking to me again.)

> *The superstrings of your life can be broken, lost or tossed away.*
>
> *Strand upon strand, they weave; though few – very few – are repeated, none are entirely without meaning.*
>
> *With time and nurture, these shoots can pierce through the singularity of the soul.*
>
> *Which is where things really get interesting.*
>
> *But wait. How should these roots be cultivated? Chance and fate – however you chose to translate karma – they play a role. So too, does choice, will and experience (though these are just another expression of karma). The old adage about shallow planting springs to mind.*
>
> *The piercing of the Singularity comes from all of the above.*

---

[4] I feel as if I should continually assert that these blog writings were the product of mania, and do not reflect my real, current, sane voice. However, after a while, these ... apologies are probably becoming just as irritating as the manic manifestos, so this will be the last one. Please take it as a given that I shift in my seat with embarrassment every time I transcribe a manic blog, or describe something ridiculous I did in my manic moments.

The hole you create– will it be a rip – a plunge – or will it be a tunnel? A wormhole, if you like: a path to a heightened reality.

For if your intellect can carry you through this long passage through the void (forget faith, that vastly weaker sibling to spirituality, for it cannot help you here), you will find the strands of your life bind together at first into an unbreakable vine (and I chose that word purposefully) where all your experience, all your choices both good and bad, become the strong cable by which you can finally carry your soul – your spirit.

Only the strong anchor of the soul can truly hoist the lesser realms of intellect, emotion, morality and the body (the latter coming last in importance), which explains why Los Angeles can be so deeply toxic for some people.

In this new space – not a void, for it is filled with love – your soul travels free, and clear, encountering other transmigrated spirits.

Your strands through the wormhole pull too, and you may be surprised who may make the passage with you given time.

He seemed to really get what I was talking about. In fact, he was probably humouring me, as I'd been humoured many times during the previous few weeks of mania; but his friendliness, and his interest in what I'd written, made me feel more human.

After I'd been in the ward for a couple of hours, it had hopefully become clear to the staff that I wasn't like the other patients. I was lucid, if grandiose, and in possession of my faculties. When I explained to them that I hadn't slept for over two nights, and couldn't sleep in my assigned room, they let me move my mattress to the music room, which they locked behind me.

During that first night, Friday night, even though I had only slept two hours since Tuesday night, I still couldn't sleep. I spent the entire night writing, striving to make sense of everything. I was still manic, and that mania drove my creativity in one huge splurge of cathartic writing. I gained new understanding of how my life path had led to this point. And this, I think, was the real value of having been locked up like this. If I'd been let free straight from the jail, I'd not have had this period of peace, where, without distraction, I could do nothing but think and write. And the result of the process was the beginnings of acceptance that I hadn't been entirely myself these past few weeks. If I hadn't been locked up, perhaps I wouldn't have accepted so soon afterwards that I was bipolar; and almost certainly there'd have been an even worse crisis, perhaps a fatal one.

By dawn, I'd written myself almost dry. I'd grouped all my various essays, poems and narratives into an eighty-page book, written in the form of a long letter to my friends. It included heartfelt apologies for what I'd put them through, but also a plea for understanding. I still held out a request for them to consider whether any of my ideas had merit, despite them having their origin in mania[5].

Saturday was another hard, long day. I now had had four days with no sleep, except for the two hours on Wednesday night. I was frequently allowed to stay locked in the music room. But they had to unlock it regularly so that the patients could play the radio, projected out of the music room window into the courtyard, where they took their smoking breaks, and, bizarrely, played basketball. It's been one of the curses of my six-foot-six height that I'm approached, almost on a daily basis, to ask if I play basketball. Each break time, I

---

[5] Fortunately, I never ended up giving this entire package of writing to Ben, or to anybody else for that matter.

held my breath with the hope that none of the patients would have the nerve to ask me.

I'd finally run out of things to write about. I was inconceivably tired but could still neither sleep, nor read, although Ben had brought me a couple of my favourite books by Patrick O'Brian, including my original copy, bought fifteen years earlier, of *Master and Commander*, a book of enormous sentimental value to me – his protagonists Aubrey & Maturin are like intimate friends to me. But it was a measure of the intensity of my feelings towards Ben and Dean that I ripped off the front cover of that book to write words meant only for them, feeling that Ben, in particular, would understand the gesture. All of my hopes for lasting through the day were focused on Ben visiting me that night, and the certainty I'd be released.

When Ben finally came that evening, we were allowed twenty minutes together, almost alone, except for the monitor, who read to himself discretely across the room. At one point, Ben stopped outside for a minute to have a word with a staff member, and I happened to notice a text on Ben's phone, a supportive note to Ben from our friends Tom and Marvin. I cried again, because it showed me not only how lucky we were with our friends, but also how much pain Ben had been through.

But the news Ben brought was terrible. There was no way around the regulations; if somebody was admitted to the system from jail as a suicide risk, then they had to be held three nights.

After Ben left, I lay on my bed in my room, feeling lost, lonely, incredibly alone. Not caring if my out-of-it roommate noticed or not, I cried on and off for the rest of the day. I cried with such facility for a man who, except for during the previous few days, hadn't cried once in well over a decade. I cried for myself, but mostly I cried for the harm I'd done to my friends and family, particularly Ben and Dean.

Finally, that Saturday night, I slept; my only sleep since the few hours on Wednesday night. On Sunday

Broken Whole

morning, I took my first shower in four days. As I came out of the shower, I looked at my now bearded face in the mirror. I stared into my eyes. And I saw ... myself. I grinned, and suddenly I knew that not only was I okay, but that I could get through the remainder of my stay. Of course, I cried again. But now they were tears of poignancy, relief and joy. I'd come back to myself.

The Green Pebble, late August

For the weeks leading up to my arrest, I'd been fixated on the idea of karma. After Ben visited me on Saturday night to tell me that I wouldn't get out until Monday, I was bitterly disappointed; but I was also exalted by a stunning, almost karmic coincidence. Monday, August 20th, would mark not only my release from the system, but also the twentieth anniversary of my arrival in the United States (or *Amerika*, as I liked to say), as a grad student. I longed to spend that night having a celebratory dinner with the two most important people in my life, Ben and Dean.

Later that Saturday night, Ben called me, and told me what he hadn't dared tell me during my visit. It wasn't even a certainty that I would get out on Monday night: they could hold me for days longer, at the discretion of the psychologist, a man I already disliked and distrusted. I was almost inconsolable. I'd wanted to surprise Ben and Dean on Monday night by telling them of the significance of the twentieth of August, 2006. Now it seemed possible I'd still be in the psychiatric system. I decided to tell Ben why it was important for me to get out on Monday, in the hope that Dean could pull extra levers. But Ben reluctantly stopped me: my dates were off. Sunday was the twentieth, not Monday, so there was no way, no matter how many levers Dean pulled, that I'd be out until at least the twenty-first. So, on the twentieth anniversary of my arrival in this country, I was in the loony bin. Supreme irony was to mark the anniversary date: so much for karma. Needless to say, I cried again.

On Monday morning, the psychiatrist gave permission for my release. My belongings were returned to me, I said goodbye to the staff members, almost all of whom had been very kind to me, and met Ben outside the locked door to the ward. I was finally free, and our lives could begin to return to normal.

Ben took the week off work, and we tried to regain some sort of routine. That Friday we even met up with a large group of friends at our regular haunting ground, the Abbey, in West Hollywood. I'd never before so much appreciated the hugs from good friends as those that I received that night. Nobody treated me any differently than usual, except for extra warmth in their embraces.

Although I'd never been a spiritual person until this summer, apart from the brief dalliance with born-again Christianity in college, my series of increasingly violent crises had taught me something very profound. My dad had also had a life-changing experience a few years earlier, when my mother, which whom he'd shared a deeply devoted love, had developed Alzheimer's. After she died my father began to open up in ways I never expected. I now knew something of what he'd gone through: I hadn't lost anybody, but I had come close to losing myself, and had gone through something that had gradually forced me to reconsider spirituality.

Shortly after my release, I was reminded that I'd come to believe that karma had merit. Ben and I were heading to brunch; as we tried to dart across the street, we were almost run over by an aggressive guy in a new black Range Rover, who swore at us through his open window (a not uncommon situation in Los Angeles). I thought to myself that karma, sooner or later, will bite him back (hopefully in the form of a black Range Rover, I'd add, if it weren't such bad karma to think so).

That day, it seemed life was starting to return to something approaching normality; we had brunch by ourselves on a beautiful Los Angeles day at Basix on Santa Monica Blvd, in West Hollywood.

As was my wont, I toyed with the green pebble I'd been keeping in my pocket ever since the day when I'd almost gone insane racing to our couples' counselling meeting. It was one of many such pebbles; they had virtually no value; in fact we had a whole bowl full of them from Pottery Barn. But this was what made the choice of the pebble a good one: I didn't need to get attached to any one particular pebble, and if we ran out I could just pop over to Pottery Barn.

By this time, I'd realized that during that one night after Ben picked me up after my "crazy" day, I'd used the word 'breathe' over and over again in my mind as a form of transcendental meditation, without realizing it. I'd tried and failed to meditate in my past; but that night meditation had found me and come to my aid. I'd also realized that when I'd placed the green pebble under my bed sheet as a painful reminder to "breathe", I'd stumbled, again out of need, upon an understanding of the use of pain in spiritual rituals. So the green pebble had come to mean a lot to me. It was the token of discovery for my own spiritual meanings.

While I fondled the pebble, my hand on the table, Ben asked me my favourite colour, probably to distract me from the endless series of thoughts and ideas still bubbling up (I was still manic, but no longer dangerously so.) I realized he'd never asked me that simple question before. I automatically answered 'blue', but really it wasn't a choice that had any true, deep meaning me: I'd always said it because my eyes were blue.

With one hand, I held Ben's hand, and, in the other, fingered the pebble. Ben had, by now, arrived at a vague understanding of how I was using it. Suddenly I paused in thought for a long time, and then spent an additional minute or two to arrange my thoughts so that I could explain to Ben what had just hit me through sense memory. Fingering the stone, I'd suddenly remembered that my dad too had had a talismanic device he always kept in his pocket, when I was a child. In his case, it was a larger, smooth, black nut that had the texture of a pebble. I'd always idly wondered what it meant to him, but had never asked him.

But now this recognition of something I had in common with my father reminded me that, with increasing frequency over the previous few weeks, I'd recognized a lot of myself in other people, and had also seen a lot of their qualities in myself. I'd wondered about it: why had I suddenly begun to see so many new similarities between myself and others? I'd never been spiritual; yet suddenly this physical connection to a simple object had shown me that I had something additional connecting me to my father. And I realized that the reason for my seeing so many similarities in others was that my mind was constantly exploring, in a manic fashion, trying to figure the world out, including its denizens: I touched upon so many different subjects in my mint, that, inevitably, there were more connection points between myself and others.

As I explained my idea about my connection to my father to Ben, a new thought came to me. I'd read a little bit about Buddhist teachings. In fact Ben, who studied philosophy in college, undoubtedly knew a lot more about it than I did. (Ironically enough, David had often mentioned the connection he'd increasingly observed between meditational or Buddhist approaches one the one hand, and cognitive therapy on the other.) My new thought was that perhaps what I had been doing in seeing this connection – the bridging of the gulf between two individuals – was the beginning of the recognition of all of our common humanity. As corny as it sounds, love for friends and family begins to spread out to a love for the world. I asked myself, and Ben, could that be what the mystics call Enlightenment?

I find myself laughing with myself as I write these sentences, since it sounds like I'm espousing the sort of gauzy, ill-defined, grasping spirituality I have always deprecated. I had ended up, after all these years, firmly in the camp of believing spirituality is something whose meaning you have to discover for yourself.

As we left the restaurant, later, Ben suddenly said, hey, if you're favourite colour is blue, what about the *Zen Room*? The Zen Room is this curious, small space in our house on which we've lavished more interior design spending than on any other room, even though we've never used it for its apparent purpose, meditation. Everything in this room is green. (I've still never used it for meditation, ever since I saw a spider in there.)

A few days later, I posted my observations about the green pebble on my blog. My sister Kirstie and her partner read the blog, and it touched me very much when Kirstie told me that that both of them were now carrying little pebbles in their pocket. And after Dean read the blog, I realized that I now had the perfect way to express to him how much he meant to me. I gave him a beautiful gift box – one that had contained one of my expensive purchases from Vuitton. Inside was a single Pottery Barn green pebble.

Messiah

After the crisis was over, it seemed a little coincidental to me, after the fact, that the first piece of music I chose to play on my car stereo, the first time I drove again (or rather, the first time Ben let me drive again), was the opening theme from the Zeffirelli production of *Jesus of Nazareth*. The music reflects a striking, painful invocation of a perceived violent rupture in space and spirituality by Jesus and his followers. I hadn't consciously chosen to play this CD for a particular reason: I'd just grabbed it on the way to the car as something different to play.

As I drove, playing it over and over again, letting the shrieking chords and the measured gravity wash over me, I found myself crying. It had not been an ostensibly deliberate choice even to buy this CD. A few months earlier, I'd recalled I used to like the soundtrack as a kid, and had ordered it on Amazon.com.

But after my reaction to playing the opening theme had passed, while I was still driving, it struck me as an entirely apt piece of music to be the first choice I made after my brush with insanity. It reminded me of the moment on my "crazy" day, when I'd been driving back to my house with Myles, when the spiritual domain had abruptly opened for me. I had been about to speak to him about Christ. It had come to me that Jesus probably never thought nor stated that he was the Son of God. Or if he had indeed made such a claim, then he was talking in a parable best calculated to have the most positive effect on those around him. I believed that he was undoubtedly one of the most spiritually alive men who had ever lived. As a result, spiritual growth had started happening around Jesus, I thought to myself. Like a pebble dropped in an infinite pond, spreading ripples ever outward, through the remainder of Jesus' short life, that effect was exponential, and had started a movement. Christ himself left no writing, so we were receiving his ideas second and third hand, in writings written decades or generations after his death, during which time his actions had been translated into terms people were more likely to accept and understand: miracles. At his death, Jesus was beaten, and subdued; yet millennia later there are magnificent buildings like Sacré Coeur dedicated to him, all because a few disciples claim they saw him alive a few days after he supposedly died on a cross. (There's a joke I heard somewhere that says if Jesus came today for the second time, he'd look at Sacré Coeur and say: 'No! That's not what I meant!')

As I was driving with Myles, and felt my mind expanding exponentially, I saw that my ideas too could spread. I thought that I was undoubtedly going to have a huge effect on people around me, but I might remain largely unknown at my death. Yet the spirituality spurred in others would sweep through those who'd known me, and perhaps they would put it into words, and a movement would begin that could change the world.

As a seven-year old, I'd expected much of myself. Yet my life had gone off track. Then, in the car with Myles, I'd suddenly wondered if I was destined to have a greater impact on the world than I could ever have conceived of as a seven-year old.

I deliberately refrained from mentioning this earlier in the book. I'd like to say that it was because I thought that without the correct context, readers might immediately abandon the book as being the writings of a self-delusional crackpot. In fact, I was nervous about putting it into writing at all, and it's not without trepidation that I admit now what I was thinking. In my manic brilliance, nothing seemed beyond my comprehension. As my intellect grew during that car ride I knew real fear: what would I grow into? I imagined that a few centuries after my death, people might have warped my teachings into a new religion. I thought it possible that I could become, in the eyes of others, a messiah; that some people, perhaps, might even see me as the Second Coming of Christ. (Note: I never thought I really *was* a Messiah – please at least give me credit for that.)

Broken Whole

Now, days after coming out of the psych ward, after listening to the soundtrack in the car, I pulled over to think. Having come through the other side of mania, I found it completely inconceivable that I could have truly thought I'd be seen as a latter day messiah. But I also thought, inevitably, of the seeming coincidence of using the metaphor of a pebble causing a ripple, given that later on in the day I'd had those messianic thoughts, and I'd used Pottery Barn green pebbles as a meditational aid to get me through the night. Then, at brunch, just after getting out of the psychiatric system, the same pebble had taught me about connectedness while I was having brunch with Ben.

Looking back, it's almost difficult, even for me, not to notice the strange repetition of the pebble motif. But I don't believe in karma really, do I? I'm a radical empiricist, aren't I?

Book IV – On Being Crazy
Back from the Brink, early September

Over the early weeks after leaving the psychiatric system, I began to slowly and painfully come to terms with the possibility I might be bipolar. I say 'possibility' deliberately, because, at first, in my ongoing manic state, I still hadn't fully conceded that the *new me* was, in total, the product of mental-illness. Despite my recent experience "in the system", I still felt full of brio and self-confidence, and my experiences of the long night of hell had reinforced the conviction that I was stronger than ever. In my view of the world, the LAPD had tried to break me and failed. When I reviewed the events of that night, I felt that I was not completely in the wrong on many points, although I also recognized that I'd been insisting on my rights to the point of self-destruction.

As the summer declined, I felt sure that, although I was probably bipolar, I'd also completely and miraculously recovered from depression. For the first time, I'd become a whole person, and fulfilled the personality I'd have owned had I not spent half my life buried in the grey mist of depression and chronic fatigue. I liked this person a lot. I was taking medication to control the mania, but all of the positive changes gained through the summer remained with me.

Although I felt I was a changed person – changed mostly for the better - I also now began to slowly recognize that a lot of my goals and ideas had been overwhelmingly grandiose. And viewing things through this prism forced me to start the process of identifying which parts of me were "the illness", and which my own, as if the two weren't the same thing.

I did, however, begin to understand the word "crazy", and even identify with it. I came across a review of a movie in the *New York Times*, a comedy – if that's possible – about a bipolar guy. The reviewer described, in a very offhand manner, the protagonist as "crazy", without seemingly being aware of the hurtful prejudice in his words. It made me recognize that the average person plainly saw mentally ill people as being almost less than fully human. Normal people – i.e. the assumed audience of the *Times*, were in a group together free and separate from the group of "crazy" people, and could feel free to not identify with them, and refer to them as if they couldn't also be a rational reader of the *Times*.

Whenever I heard the word 'crazy' bandied about like that, I'd have a sudden feeling of disassociation to realize afresh that it was possible to lump me into that category. I wasn't, apparently, in the self-defined "normal" group of *Times* readers, even though I'd been reading the *Times* daily for two decades and felt I was a card carrying member. So it was possible that others viewed me as crazy, with all the scary connotations of that word.

The full meaning of "crazy" took weeks to sink in, but there was a distinct moment when I suddenly understood something very important. When I'd been on the edge of losing my sanity that day on the streets of Hollywood, and had barged into a 7-11, and had poured my bottle of tequila over the counter to force the clerk to call 911, the witnesses, including the kind young gay guy who tried to help me, must have seen me as a crazy guy. I was definitely not behaving normally, and obviously needed help. If I'd seen similar behaviour, I'd have thought the same. We all come across "crazy" people regularly, or, at least, you do if you live in a major city. Most homeless people seem to have a mental illness, and we hear them talking to themselves, or shouting out loud at the world. The very strange thing is that when I poured the tequila on the counter at 7-11, I was behaving in what was to me a completely rational manner, given what I was going through. Something had gone physically wrong in my brain, and the only way I knew to save myself was to get tranquilized. It felt inconceivably urgent. That's why I'd taken, by force, the tequila from the bar on Sunset – to self-medicate. I knew, with almost complete certainty, that if I didn't receive medical attention soon I might be swept away in the maelstrom inside my head, possibly permanently, and I did whatever it took to get help.

There seems to be an impenetrable barrier between what a "normal" person sees, and what a mentally ill person feels, although both are witnesses to the same event, which, in my case, was the internal meltdown. I, myself, need to remind myself of this when I see a street person on the street. You see, just as I don't walk around with the constant knowledge that I'm what some people might describe as freakishly tall, I also don't walk around thinking to myself, gee, I'm crazy. I identify, instead, with the "normal" *New York Times* readers. The street people I see may themselves know, as I did, that they are obviously seriously off kilter, and probably appear crazy. Yet in their minds, they may have entirely rational reasons for doing whatever it is that makes people think they're crazy.

The first difficult encounter after my release was with my psychiatrist. I had only a very short (scandalously short, in retrospect) appointment with her. One of the things she was worried about was the flight of ideas and agitation. Yet who could expect me to explain these two crazy weekends in ten minutes, without sounding agitated? It was a crazy request. So I duly got agitated, and a glazed look entered her eyes as I saw that I'd not only lost her, but also confirmed, in her mind, her own hypothesis. Although the meeting didn't go well, I did agree to keep taking the anti-psychotic medication I'd been prescribed in the psychiatric ward.

Ever since Dallas, where I'd begun to see evidence of explosive intellectual growth, I'd been intending to see Dr. Serpa, a clinical neuropsychologist, to get a full battery of IQ tests. I was sure I'd be well past genius level. On the day Myles was driving me home, just before I had my crazy half hour on the streets of Hollywood, I'd felt that I could poke my mind into every nook and cranny of creation. I still wonder, to this day, was I truly super intelligent at that moment? The mind is a curious and misunderstood organ. For myself, I stick to my empirical conclusion that a manic mind is capable of brilliance. I did have some piercing, life-changing insights while I was manic. But where the manic mind falls down is on winnowing the brilliant ideas from the crazy and unrealistic ones. If you're looking for examples, look no further than my belief that a (fraudulent) solution to endless customer-service voice menus could change the world economy.

Shortly after seeing my psychiatrist, I finally managed to get an appointment with Serpa. He was an extremely kindly, sympathetic man, with an office in a small, beautiful building in West Hollywood. His office was, of all things, painted green, and I felt immediately at home with him. He gave me plenty of time to explain what had happened over the last few weeks, culminating in the jail crisis.

After hearing me out, he asked me what medication I was taking. I told him the dosages of Seroquel, Abilify and Depakote that I was taking. This became the turning point for me, the point at which it began to come home to me that I was indeed bipolar, and that it was a condition I'd have to live with for the rest of my life. He told me that any normal person taking those levels of those drugs would not be, as I was right then, full of energy and vitality, but would be, instead, practically asleep on the couch. He said that he wouldn't agree to give me the IQ tests just now, but that if I still felt that I needed them after I'd stabilized on my medications, he'd reconsider.

The next morning, I told Ben that I was ready to admit I was bipolar.

Okay, So I'm Bipolar. Now What?

For any bipolar person, the first manic episode is the most difficult. All those around you can recognize there is something terribly wrong, but you yourself have no experience of mania to draw upon, and are in the midst of something that seems wondrous and empowering. I'd thought of myself as this huge, violently hued flower unfurling unexpectedly, attracting all with its colour and grandeur. My friends, on the other hand, had smelled the rotting core. I'd felt that I was coming into the light for the first time in over twenty years; inheriting my full self, a self that had charm, charisma, creativity, intelligence and self-confidence; a self that could accomplish almost anything. But I'd failed to see the grandiosity, and impossibility of many of my ideas, and hadn't listened to those like Dean and Ben who'd tried to slow me down. In fact I'd accused Dean of a lack of trust, and Ben of over-anxiety.

My first (and only) major manic episode lasted many months, beginning in San Diego. It had been triggered by taking Lexapro, and then massively boosted by the week of hellish stress in Dallas. After that it had taken on a life of its own. It had peaked on the night I was arrested, and then, once I began to take medication, began to wane. But it took as long to wane as it did to build, so, for weeks after I was released from the psychiatric ward, I was still manic. The difference was that I now knew I was manic; and I'd seen how terribly destructive it had been both to myself and my friends and family. I felt I could control and master it.

But that didn't mean that the mania-fuelled creativity went away. And I found – quite naturally, I suppose – that people were still worrying about me. It became extremely painful. I felt I'd finally earned the right to talk about some of my business ideas with enthusiasm and conviction. My friends and family would sound excited on the phone or in person, yet they'd later say to Ben that I didn't sound myself, or that they were worried. I felt very betrayed and hurt. 'Of course I'm not the same person,' I wanted to yell at them! 'Who can go through what I went through and be the same person? If you don't want to hear my ideas, just tell me to shut up! Don't say, wow, that sounds exciting, and then privately talk about me behind my back as if you think I'm crazy. I don't want to cut you out of my ideas!'

At the beginning of my long manic phase during the summer, I'd actually stopped reading the *New York Times* entirely. I'd been working seventeen-hour days, and barely sleeping, so I'd had to prioritize. Given the choice between reading the *Times*, and working out at the gym, I was always going to choose the latter. Or at least that had felt like the reason for my dropping the *Times* from my daily schedule. Similarly, I'd stopped running, for the first time in years. I'd even stopped biting my nails (not, in this case, because I didn't have time, but because – presumably – whatever anxiety drove me to bite my nails was in abeyance.)

But the change I noticed the most was that my life-long habit of reading in bed before sleep was becoming problematic. I'd barely got through *Parallel Worlds* by Michio Kaku, the astounding book on cosmology which had given me so many wild ideas; and I'd not even been able to focus on my old friends Aubrey and Maturin, the dual protagonists in Patrick O'Brian's twenty-book-long series of naval historical fiction. If I was reading something I was already too familiar with, the ideas from the day would intrude. On the other hand, more challenging reading could be over stimulating, and could keep me awake for hours. So I found I had to read material right in the middle. Which proved to be *Star Trek* novels.

Although I'd been a life-long fan of *Star Trek*, I'd never read many novels. I've always been something of an elitist in my reading choices, never reading what I considered low-brow fiction such as thrillers or *Star Trek* novels. Or *Harry Potter*. But now I discovered, to my amazement, that the *Star Trek* novels by William Shatner (and co-authors) were really quite good. They contained strong science-fiction ideas, and an utter familiarity with characters I'd grown to love: in other words, it was just enough to keep my mind from taking up ideas I'd generated during the day, but not enough to generate new ones (although I did start to plot a *Star Trek* novel of my own.)

When sleep still wouldn't come, I'd resort to reading fluffy but expensive fashion and interior design magazines. I'd cut out and file ideas for travel, tech gadgets, home, and especially hot outfits. (One of the more interesting symptoms shown by manic people is dressing "far more flamboyantly and colourfully than they would normally do". Oh Lord, some of the things I wore when I was under the influence of mania.) Eventually, some combination of prescription drugs and alcohol would gradually slow down my thoughts enough to allow sleep to steal upon me.

Now, once I knew I was bipolar, the truth of coming to terms with it, and also with the flux of creativity that continued, meant that it truly *was* dangerous to expose myself to too many ideas. As Reverend Beebe says in *A Room with a View*, 'I put it down to too much Beethoven.' In my case, it was too much Zarathustra. Almost anything could trigger a set of associations that would lead me into uncharted territory. One of my favourite pieces of classical music – in fact one of the (if not the most) most dramatic pieces of all classical music – was *Also Sprach Zarathustra*, the half-hour tone poem by Richard Strauss, the beginning of which is most familiarly known as the opening theme from *2001 a Space Odyssey*. While listening to it one day in the car, it struck me as a perfect piece of music to describe what I'd been through. By this time, I'd been writing my blog for a few weeks, and I'd used the analogy of a singularity exploding into the Big Bang, in a blog titled *An Encounter with the Void*, to describe the transformative experience I'd been through. Now, listening to it in the car, when I heard the opening of "Zarathustra", I suddenly recognized that it was an approach to understanding the *encounter with the void*. It was this perfect piece of whole music – blasting at you as you approach the singularity. But once you're through the wormhole at the centre of the void (I extended the analogy), you dither and float around in the wake of the void, much like the music that follows the opening fanfare, which sounds as if it's completely lost its footing (much to the disappointment of unforewarned symphony audiences everywhere). It was a very fanciful analogy, I realized; but it seemed so important to me at the time that I installed the opening of "Zarathustra" as the ring-tone on my cell-phone. Ben showed incredible patience with having to listen to my ridiculously tiny cell-phone (especially for my large hands) banging out the timpani on its tinny speakers.

An Encounter with the Void goes like this:

> *On Friday, I touched the void. I felt the very blood of time pulsing against my fevered forehead. The path that preceded the void was precipitous. I scared passers-by, and almost toyed with them, as I realized how powerful I'd become. I scorched past fame, riches and celebrity barely long enough to recognize them. Intellectuality, more cunningly appealing, held me in its grasp a lot longer, for its roots were much more entrenched. Indeed, it alone ultimately carried me unharmed through the void. But in the path to the void, I said and did things both which I now regret, and which played a role in the journey. I entertained chilling ideas and felt I could understand God.*

> *There was only one true path to the void fated for me, and that was via love. When love tightened its hold on me that Friday afternoon, I spun off inconceivably rapidly, fell headlong towards the Singularity, and was caught suspended inches from Chaos, swinging by the narrow thread of my intellect. For half an hour I became thoroughly acquainted with the Singularity, until moment by moment I began*

to realize I could save love only by saving myself first. I clawed painfully, haltingly up the thread, yet feeling the pull of the void, and slipping back a few inches now and again.

When Ben arrived to rescue me, I finally knew the void had lost its pull on me for good, and indeed have no longer that fear.

My intellect too survived and flourished, leading me through the rest of that awful day, as I discovered the overarching concept of karma.

You can never be the same, once you've survived the void, and to many you may appear irretrievably altered. And you may still bounce around in the wake of the void for days, weeks or months before you again find true peace.

By entertaining fanciful ideas, though, I was getting myself into dangerous territory. The day after my first *Zarathustra* apotheosis, I had lunch with Ben at UCLA, and decided to grab a copy of *Also Sprach Zarathustra*, the original philosophical text which inspired the music, to see if my interpretation of the opening section of the music had anything to do with Nietzsche's philosophy. As I was driving home down Wilshire Boulevard, I skimmed the introduction to get an understanding of the basic thesis of the book. Almost immediately, a flood of ideas followed for a blog article, none of which had anything to do with my original analogy about the music. Once I was in the flats of Beverly Hills, I kept pulling over to scribble my thoughts down, and when I got home, hastily wrote and posted the article on my blog.

I titled my new blog entry *Übermensching Nietzsche*. It was only after I'd posted it that I realized the date was September 11th, 2006, five years since 9/11. (Dramatic coincidences like that seem to abound to the manic.) So I added the subtitle: *Or why can't we all just get a bit of 9/11?*

> *... Nietzsche's central thesis seems, to me, to be that we all have to go through a near-death experience if we're to change into an Überman, and hence have a positive effect on the world.*

> *... I don't know what the answer is. It has to be something that simultaneously changes us all along the Zarathustra lines. It need not be a near-death experience. Look at Bill Gates for example (who now realizes he has the power to change the world through philanthropy). But it seems that near-death is the most likely thing to do it, although I doubt even a near death experience would do anything to change Dick Cheney into something resembling a human being.*

> *But for it to have a critical mass, we probably all need to have a near death experience together. It seems to me that Steven Spielberg and Star Trek got it right. In both "Close Encounters of the Third Kind", and "Star Trek: First Contact", the first contact with a benevolent alien civilization was enough. It was, in neither case, a near death experience, which is why I'd go further, and say it does not need to be a malevolent encounter. So long as we can overcome our collective encounter with the void, we'll be okay going forward.*

This is a good example of the perspective shift experienced in mania. While manic, I could write about *Zarathustra*, and even criticize it, believing I'd had a fresh insight worth sharing with the world. A few days later, my essay was posted on *gayspirituality.com*, and I received a comment from a *real* philosopher making it clear that I'd misread Nietzsche. And so embarrassed reality hit: how could I have conceivably thought that I could understand such a complex philosophical book – not to mention postulate an original meaning – with five minutes of reading and no serious background in philosophy? It was a similar mistake, albeit on a much smaller scale, to the manic discovery that precipitated my brush with insanity. It's impossible, once you come down from a manic high, to put yourself back in the head of the person who had those thoughts. There were many such smaller self-delusions over the slow decline of mania in the fall, some of which I'm ashamed, even now, to write about.

My realization that listening to the music had led to buying the book, which, in turn, had led me to excitedly driving while philosophizing, drove home to me that I was still manic. In this case the results had been relatively harmless. But I knew, from the experiences of the previous few weeks of crises, where sudden ideas could lead me. I made the firm decision to temporarily cut out my life anything that was overly intellectually stimulating: no art movies, no deep conversations with friends or acquaintances, and, most importantly, no serious reading. After all, there were many more bad *Star Trek* novels to read.

But things kept happening, despite my best efforts to keep my life simple. It seemed almost everything was capable of stimulating my mind. One day, I popped *Crime of the Century*, by Supertramp, into the DVD player in the car. I hadn't listened to it in years. As I drove, I found myself whistling along to the music, using my lips and vocal chords simultaneously for syncopation, until ... I abruptly ceased as I realized that enthusiastic whistling to music in the car (something I used to do all the time) is yet another activity that could make me feel slightly manic.

And there were the dangers inherent in having an extremely outgoing, intellectual boyfriend whose mind could range freely on an almost infinite number of topics. Our intellectual curiosity was part of the glue that held our relationship together, and we'd often been used to having exciting conversations at the breakfast table. But now, I found that these conversations could start my head buzzing, literally as if an electric current was running through my cranium.

(As I write this, Ben is sitting across the dining-room table from me, and has just been telling me about the controversy on a paper he's been trying to submit for publication. He talks with such animation, his broad forehead reddening and furrowing, and his eyes gleaming, that anybody watching would think … well … that he's a maniac.)

It wasn't even safe for me to do absolutely nothing, since then my mind would be at its most active, sparking randomly in all directions. One night at home, I was doing something very rare – relaxing. I was attempting to practice mindfulness, and just lay there, doing nothing but listening and looking – really looking – at things. Our living room has an aura of calm at night. There are usually no sounds except an occasional ching-toom from the wind-chime on our balcony. Pools of light on a red rug and the iridescent red table-runners on the dining room table; the green glow from a beautiful standing lamp; the comfort of a chic Italian sofa made of green leather with espresso wood fixtures: it's a place to escape from the world; it's a place associated with the comfort of my relationship with Ben.

I could get into this relaxation thing, I thought, and decided to make some *Sleepy-Time* tea, with its calming medley of chamomile and peppermint – a harmless, innocuous activity, right? I boiled water in our bright red metal kettle, which in itself provided a few seconds of beauty, sounding a double-note mellifluous tone when the water boiled.

I was pouring the water into the pot when: bam! The idea hit. Why not write a blog about this whole process of relaxation? And we were off! A sudden flurry of other ideas all jumping up and down, wanting to be included in the blog, trying to climb into the tea pot and drown out the one good idea with their clamouring voices. Inside of a minute of the idea hitting, my mind was buzzing.

After scribbling the main points down, I deliberately said a stern 'No!' to the remainders, leaving them scrambling at the door to my conscious mind. I poured a cup of tea, and returned to the sofa, picking up the *New York Times*, feeling good that I hadn't let the ideas steal the show. There were no noises except the wind-chime, and the endless peeps emanating from the squeaky toy rabbit that our little puppy could enjoy for hours at a stretch, days without end. I wondered what it must be like to be amused by just one idea at a time. That thought gave me more ideas for my blog, and I virtually ran into my office and laid hands on the keyboard, all ideas of mindfulness and peace left behind in the living room, along with the tea.

Shortly after I got out of hospital, we spent a quiet "recovery" weekend in Palm Springs, staying with Bill and Stephane. I was still glowing with self-confidence, and flush with bonhomie, despite my experiences. On Saturday night, Ben and I walked into Hunters, a popular gay club, where, by chance, the "Mr. Gay Palm Springs" competition was taking place. The very minute we walked through the door of the club, the organizer was in my face, good-naturedly demanding that I sign myself up as a last minute entrant. I was in the best shape of my life after two months of manic energy, and it was fun to take part in the silliness. Every time I had to go on stage, I got to see Ben's huge grin, easily visible despite the glare of the spotlights; but I really didn't care whether I won or not. I was a good sport about it, but when they wanted everybody to go on stage wearing ugly boxers, I declined, and just wore my jeans instead. The nail in the coffin for my chances of winning the competition, however, was my extemporaneous speech.

'I'm really not here to win the competition. A few weeks ago I almost resigned my job. A week later I almost went insane. Two weeks after that I was in jail. So I'm just here to have fun.'

With that, I handed the microphone back to the drag-queen emcee, who looked first at me and then at the crowd with a forced, perplexed smile.

Despite trying to close myself off to new sources of stimulation, I had no intention of giving up some of the better ideas I'd come up with during the peak of my mania. My main focus was on following up with the idea of starting *Club Karma*: now, however, I'd narrowed down the concept significantly to being just a new monthly event starting off with a much smaller promotional event.

I still believed there were no problems I could not solve. The customer service idea that had precipitated my brush with insanity had not gone away. Not long after the crisis on the streets of Hollywood, after I'd bought the domain name customerserviceanytime.com and had incorporated under that name, I paid $5,000 to a web-design company to create my online presence, dominated by a yellow logo wrapped around a rubber duck (don't ask). I still fancied the plan would work, and imagined that I'd start off as the sole problem solver behind the scenes, and would tackle literally any customer-service issue faced by a consumer, for a fee.

I felt incredibly centred, with an unwavering, or so I thought, moral compass. I never failed to recognize and try to right injustices, even intervening in a fight in a gay bar, holding one of the brawlers at bay. Yet, in some ways I remained strangely blind: it took me several weeks to realize that the central tenet of my customer service idea was fraudulent, even if well-intentioned, since it involved lying to companies in order to reach people deep in the organization under false pretenses (that is, impersonating a well-known reporter from the New York Times.)

At the same time, I had several ideas for writing books (including the *Star Trek* novel), and large ambitions for the future of my blog. I still, secretly, believed that wealth and fame were just around the corner. If all else failed, there were always the damages I expected to win against the Omni Hotel and the LAPD.

I was very careful, though, not to worry Ben about the pursuit of my ideas; I tried to stop myself doing the things that had scared him most when I was manic. For instance, I suppressed, albeit with some difficulty, more cheerful engagement with strangers, and tried not to make as many notes in my ever-present mania-purchased Montblanc pocket note-book, or my new pocket digital recorder. This last promise became a particularly difficult one to keep when I started to develop this book, so when we were working out together at the gym, I'd vanish around the corner and surreptitiously voice a few notes.

For all my ideas, I was no longer acting dangerously upon them. After briefly contemplating spending the $5,000 on P.R., I'd cut off my spending completely, because I'd had to accept I was in a serious financial situation - the worst of my life: during my manic period I'd accumulated an additional $80,000 of debt on various store cards and credit cards.

There were, however, fresh things to conceal from Ben, and he's about to read of some of them here for the first time (as I write, it's three years on from the summer of 2006.) Ben had already been shocked at the extent of my shopping, and yet he never saw all of it. After things had come to a head, I'd been so ashamed of my spending that I rented a very small storage space near LAX in which to hide some of the clothing I hadn't told Ben about. It was only a handful of things; all of them very nice and flattering. (I wish I could have kept them.) I tried to sell them on *eBay*, and then, after that failed, through special consignment in a high-end thrift store. But that fell through too. (It was, after all, rather hard to find a slim, broad-shouldered, 6'6 guy who was comfortable wearing such extravagant clothing.), I finally stuffed them into a paper bag and dumped them in a trash can on Santa Monica Boulevard.

Even today, in 2009, as I was driving with Ben doing our usual Saturday chores, something else came out. When I was in the midst of developing my plans for Karma, I'd attempted to rope in both friends and strangers. For instance, my friend Cecilia had always wanted to open a wine bar, and I added that idea into the mix for the club, along with a coffee shop, a gallery, fashion shows, and décor which included exotic mannequins. This is what just came out today while driving with Ben, when he noticed the startlingly original mannequins created by a young kid who works in a local thrift store we visited today. I off-handedly told him that I knew the kid who made them, and, when he asked why, sheepishly admitted that I'd asked him to do décor for my club. The manic period was so intense, that there were a million such ideas and stray thoughts, actions, conversations, and promises, most of the details of which I've since forgotten about, but some of which come, every now and then, back into memory. Many people – those who didn't know me – where only too glad to be drawn in, including a bipolar girl who worked at D&G in the Beverly Center who encouraged me to buy their entire line of sailor-inspired gear, some of which ended up in that trash-can on Santa Monica Blvd.

I had a lot of time to think about everything that had happened. I'd drawn my own empirical conclusion that mania magnifies your strongest personality traits: in my case, impatience, and a tendency not to let things pass. Fortunately, I'd never been a mean person, or else I'd have more than likely become violent and vicious. In my case, I'd hurt myself and Ben, and, in neither case, intentionally.

I resolutely retained the belief that I'd been in the right during both the encounter at the Ramada, and the subsequent fiasco at the Omni Hotel. As my sister Sally said, when I told her what had happened, it was that pigheadedness running through our family. I've never been, by nature, a person who enjoys confrontation, despite the fact that my dad's advice on how to handle a difficult situation at school always involved using the fist. Yet I've always been helplessly drawn to confrontation because of that Adams trait of not sitting still until wrongs are righted. I got into a lot of fights at school, either for myself or in defending a smaller friend, despite being a hopeless fighter. I could never just give face and back off.

This time, though, that same stubbornness had got me into deep waters, and, through those four awful nights in jail and then the psychiatric system, I'd realized that my mania had blinded me to something even more important than having my sense of right and wrong validated: the love of my friends and family. I'd put them through hell just to prove myself right in relatively trivial situations.

For almost all my life, my worries about my body image had been first and foremost in forming me. After that in importance, had come my intellect and my striving to form intimate friendships. The concept of the soul had always been dead last. But the summer had sent me through the wormhole, upending everything: my self-esteem was no longer controlled by whatever somebody thought of my body. After getting out of the psychiatric ward, I vowed to myself that I was always going to put the love of my friends and family first, a long, long way above getting my sense of justice validated: but, also, ahead of body; ahead of intellect too; and yes, even ahead of what I'd come to find in myself through this crisis: my soul.

Broken Whole

Ben Again

I will never be able to fathom the depths of strength Ben drew on to get us through the crisis. The combination of his personal history, along with my own newly forceful personality massively boosted by mania, was potent stuff. Anybody would be challenged by being with a life-partner experiencing his first manic episode; but Ben had been down this road before. Three years into his previous relationship – which ultimately had lasted nine years – his boyfriend, Scott, had been diagnosed with bipolar disorder. Scott hadn't had my advantages of an introspective nature and years of therapy: he didn't possess the skills to manage his own condition; that lot had fallen upon Ben, and he'd coped with it for as long as he could. Now he had to deal with it all over again.

It was still a daily battle of trust between us. We had to relearn almost everything we thought we knew about each other. Back just a few months earlier, I was still suffering from chronic depression, and was consequently inordinately sensitive, and Ben would have to worry about not upsetting me. Meanwhile, I'd do Ben's introspection for him, since he wasn't, by nature, a man who surveyed his own thought processes objectively. Now, however, I wanted to pursue my dreams without feeling like Ben was breathing down my neck. In other words, now *I* had to be the one to worry about upsetting the other person. Ben, meanwhile, had become pensive, withdrawn and battle shy. He'd always been the most happy-go-lucky, cheerful person I'd ever known; somebody who fell asleep almost as soon as his head hit the pillow. Now, he looked lost in thought all the time, and, at breakfast, I'd raise my eyes from the *New York Times* to see him just staring blankly at his *L.A. Times* without reading, his mind elsewhere. And he was taking Xanax and a glass of port (drinking from a most delicate, "girly" cup, about which I ribbed him) to get to sleep.

The antagonist remained my yearning to act upon my ideas. I felt I was finally in the light: completely free of depression and able to pursue almost limitless opportunities. But that's where our psyches clashed badly: I was used to seeing occasional expressions of anxiety from Ben, who'd, in fact, always had the tendency to worry about small things. So when Ben had, early on during the manic episode, stated his worries about the magnitude of my ideas, I'd just irritatedly scolded him for being overly anxious. Ben had begun to realize that his worries were pushing me away; whereas I'd felt he was trying to pour cold water on my grand plans. Ben had been faced with the awful choice of either holding his tongue – potentially giving me reign to ruin myself – or trying to rein me in at the risk of pushing me away.

Until the ultimate crisis, when I was arrested, I'd known that I was hurting Ben, as well as Dean and other friends, but couldn't stop myself. I was on the verge of fulfilling my selfhood, and I wasn't going to let anybody hold me back.

In the weeks of declining mania after my release from the psychiatric ward, Ben and I began to mend these fences, and spent a lot of time with our various mental health providers, both alone and together. As bad as things had been for me, I knew that it had also been a summer of hell for Ben: not just the weeks of anxiety, but also my time in jail, and then the psychiatric system. Ben had spent hours with the LAPD trying to get me released, and then both Dean and he had had to track down our car – impounded by the LAPD from the Omni Hotel – and drive it home and unpack my belongings, seeing, for the first time, the truly shocking amount of shopping I'd done in the few hours between moving out of our house and getting kicked out of the Ramada. They also had to call the W Hotel in San Francisco and cancel my month-long reservation of a corner suite.

Ben and I had already reached a point, before my manic episode, where we were able to communicate with each other clearly, but it hadn't always been easy for Ben, who, having grown up in Singapore, had been initially averse to the whole idea of therapy. It turned out to be one of the greatest blessings that I'd insisted on us getting a couples counsellor when I moved down to LA to live with him two years previously. We ended up with the kind, skillful therapist, Paul Kundinger, who probably played the biggest role, amongst our support network, in saving our relationship.

Ben had permanently absorbed a large portion of debt I'd incurred during my summer of manic spending. He told me that he'd forgiven me for this; that the matter was closed. But I began to notice that whenever an issue came up about which of us should pay for something, he'd bring up the issue of the debt that he'd paid. Ironically, in my own therapy sessions with David, I'd been used to hearing that my spending had been a symptom of the illness, and that I shouldn't feel too much guilt about it. (In case you're wondering, "manic spending" is *not* covered by most health insurance policies, which seems a little unfair since it's included in the DSM IV as a symptom.)

I brought up the issue of my financial (not to mention moral) debt to Ben in couples' therapy with Paul one day; it was beginning to seem to me that Ben hadn't really forgiven me the debt after all. He was still holding it against me.

In the meeting, skillfully led by Paul, I suggested that what really underlay Ben's actions was that I'd never fully acknowledged to him that I understood how much pain I'd put him through. Before Ben could react, an even more powerful realization swept through me, and I tried to give voice to it. In these few weeks after the crisis, I'd felt that I'd gone through a hell of suffering. I'd been the one who was sick, after all. But now I suddenly recognized that it may well have been, after all, worse for Ben than for me: much worse. He'd had absolutely no control over what was happening. I, on the other hand, had enjoyed the sheer high of mania for weeks on end, punctuated by periods of extremity. For months, there had been no escape for Ben from intense anxiety.

For the first time I approached the precipice of comprehending how Ben must have felt during these weeks, and I was swamped with a level of compassion and sorrow that I knew could overwhelm me unless I stepped back from the precipice and took my time to comprehend its entirety. I now saw that Ben had been the anchor keeping us together.

The barriers between us were suddenly broken: because I'd come to these realizations myself while speaking, uninterrupted, in therapy, Ben could see that it was unpremeditated, and that I really, finally, now understood what he'd been through. Things between us would take a long time to return to normal; but there was never any question, again, going forward, about our common forgiveness and understanding.

During the weeks since my manic peak, I'd been finding out who I really was, as had everybody else: my real self had been hidden underneath depression all these years, only peaking out now and then. My manic self, who I'd felt at times was just a magnification of my real self, had been temporarily unleashed during the summer, and was now medicated and resolving into clarity. And this clear version was pretty terrific, I thought; everything I'd always wanted to be: still burning bright, fearless, empathic, creative, and self-confident. This new version, free of depression, was difficult, in other words, to distinguish from the intensely manic version.

The experiences had left us both permanently changed. We had to renegotiate our entire relationship. We understood and trusted each other more than ever before, and yet we found ourselves arguing almost all the time. One of our worst arguments illustrated the ongoing clash between Ben's anxieties and my continuing desire to shield him from worry. The argument started with sex. Both Ben and I secretly wanted to have sex, but because of a perfect storm of a misunderstanding, Ben almost ended up having a nervous breakdown instead.

Broken Whole

That evening, in the goal of building my online photography portfolio, I'd done a shoot with Nick, a gorgeous, young Peruvian friend, whose boyfriend was in an MTV reality show, *Nemesis*. During the shoot, I was strictly professional, even while Nick lay shirtless on the bed in our guest room, his lean, muscular torso sprayed with water, and his puppy brown eyes staring soulfully at me. Ben kept darting downstairs and asking if he could be the designated spritzer.

We hadn't had sex together all week, and without discussing it, we'd both secretly wanted to have sex that night. After Nick left, Ben was working on his computer, as he does frequently, being a busy man in charge of a research lab. Or at least I thought he was working. He was actually looking at homoerotic photos online to get turned on. Meanwhile, I was retouching the photos of Nick, and planned to show them to Ben as a prelude to sex.

Both our secret plans were moving towards completion: I finished the photos, and started up the shower, which Ben took as the signal I'd be coming to bed soon. Just at that moment the plans got derailed: I suddenly had a series of ideas to improve my plan for the promotional event for Karma. I switched off the shower, and returned to my office to sketch them out.

Fifteen minutes later, Ben came into my office. He'd heard me start, then stop the shower, and came simply to ask me when I was coming to bed. But I instantly misinterpreted the look on his face as being anxiety: he was worrying, I felt, that the old, manic, note-taking Keith had returned. I looked up at him in irritation, my eyes red-rimmed from two hours of working on Nick's photos. Were all my actions to be interpreted as manic? Wasn't I allowed to be creative, I thought to myself angrily?

I explained to him vehemently that I needed just a few minutes. But, to Ben it really did look like mania all over again. He thought he could see it in my eyes. He retreated.

A few minutes later I came into the bathroom, saw his extremely worried face, and could tell what was going through his mind. He later told me that in those first moments after he'd left my office, he'd panicked, and had almost fled to go and stay with a friend. This fairly broke my heart. Ben, I saw now, was clearly suffering from post-traumatic stress: almost any trigger could take him back into the months of fear he'd endured while I was screaming towards a peak of mania.

Would we ever get back to normality? I hoped so. Ben had to learn to distinguish between the new über-Keith, and the manic Keith; I had to learn to be more sensitive towards his anxieties. It was easy enough for me to say that I wished Ben would just return to being the old Ben – the Ben who was frequently too preoccupied with his medical research to notice what I was doing. But then Ben couldn't say that he wished I could return to the old Keith, because neither of us knew who that old Keith was, nor who the new Keith would turn out to be, once he reached a point of stability.

Broken Whole

Male Model, late September

In late September, I finally got around to something I'd been meaning to try for a few weeks. I went to a cold-call at Next Model Management, in Beverly Hills. A dash of my intrinsic self-consciousness might have come in useful as I'd dressed that morning, since I was dressed in high manic style, the sort of look only somebody who was wildly self-confident could (but shouldn't) pull off.

When I arrived, there was nobody in the waiting room apart from a severe-looking receptionist, who wordlessly took my head-shots. I sat and began to write a new blog entry, to pass the time, not nervous in the least.

> *The physicality of my body has been, until very recently, the most formative issue in my life. Not that I'm handicapped in any obvious way; but somebody can be physically and mentally handicapped for almost their whole adult life while looking entirely normal, even healthy and handsome.*
>
> *I thought that this would be the appropriate time and place to start writing this blog entry, as I sit in the waiting room for a small cattle-call in one of the top modelling agencies in the world, at the age of forty-one, waiting to see if I'm about to be "discovered."*
>
> *I'm six-foot-six, a lean and muscular two-hundred-and-fifteen pounds, wearing G-star jeans, a J. Lindberg belt, and a very tight-fitting Miu-Miu black shirt, with my sleeves rolled up to the biceps, and three buttons unfastened revealing a couple of necklaces nestling against my spray-tanned chest. My mid-brown hair is spiked, and highlighted in blond. I'm carrying an expensive, Italian, brown-leather bag lined on one side with dappled fur. My Alexander*

McQueen gold skeleton key-chain is dangling by my side.

My face is a study in the years I've lived, the experiences I've been through: it's a strong face I think: good jaw line and cheek bones, full lips, and wide, deep-set blue-green eyes, surely betraying good humour and self-confidence. I've never felt more whole in my life.

Since my late twenties, I've been told many times that I should be a model. During these past few weeks, I was told it almost daily, as I flitted about the high places of West Hollywood and Beverley Hills, chasing my dreams. I'm here to see if this particular dream is for real, or can I put this ghost to rest? So, waiting, I sit here composedly writing these very words in the leather-bound writing book I bought in Dallas way back at the beginning of the explosion that marked the summer of my forty-first year.

I looked up as a harried-looking male employee popped his head into the waiting room and called my name.

I gathered my things and went through with him to the anteroom. I saw that he had my head-shots in his hands. He made a show at looking through them.

'Sorry,' he said. 'We're going to pass.'

I was curious to know the reason why.

'I'm too tall, right?' I asked.

'Yes,' he said. 'But also too edgy. If you toned your look down a bit, maybe one of the other agencies would be interested for lifestyle work.'

I smiled and thanked him. Once I was outside of the building I grinned. I checked myself inside for any sense of harm or loss, and found none. I'd been physically rejected; something that would have deeply hurt me at any earlier time in my life. Yet now I could see that not a shred of my sense of self was in any way diminished.

I had my answer at last, about modelling, and I felt a sense of freedom. As I realized that it didn't hurt me in the least to get rejected as a model, I was confirmed in my belief that what I'd learned at San Diego gay pride was true: my inner sense of self worth was no longer dependent on how people assessed my looks. I picked up my car and drove over to Skewers, a restaurant in West Hollywood, and continued writing my blog entry, sitting at one of the tables outside on Santa Monica Boulevard.

I was still mildly manic, which meant that my mind was still privy to unique, powerful, and sometimes misconceived insights that I'd most likely have missed under normal brain function. And it was this facility that suddenly shook me to the core as I lifted the pen from the paper. Out of the blue, I understood what had always eluded me: why I left kindergarten happy and gregarious, and re-emerged in grade school, only weeks later, as a shy, friendless boy. It all came together in my mind. And there was more. I now knew everything else: why I'd grown to hate myself, and consider myself unlikable, and why I'd suffered chronic mental and physical depression for most of my adult life. All of this understanding had come to me in a single flash of insight.

Many times during therapy, over the years, I'd speculated that it could have been an incident concerning my appearance. It was the very last day of kindergarten, the beginning of the summer before I arrived at my new school with a totally different personality. I was feeling the nostalgia and excitement of leaving a school where I'd been well-liked, and had been head of my class. Even at that tender age, I already knew that I found boys attractive, but I hadn't connected it with the barely understood concept of homosexuality. Nonetheless, I had lots of what I liked to call "girl-friends," all of whom I imagined crying at my departure.

That night of leaving school, with the long North Sea summer twilight stealing horizontally through our windows and the blackbirds singing through the open windows, I dashed into the bathroom, eager to wash and then go to play outside with my friends. I slipped and fell backwards; the back of my head banged against the bathroom wall propelling me violently forwards into the rim of the bathtub. The impact was directly on my front teeth, which were knocked into a horizontal position, pointing at the back of my throat. I shrieked with pain, and heard my parents bounding up the stairs.

My dad straightened my teeth with his own hands while I stood over the sink, my mouth pouring blood. I was driven in a neighbour's car to the local clinic, where all they could do was to pack my mouth with gauze. I lay in bed all night, unable to sleep. The next day I had the first of a series of visits to a dentist's office full of grimy old fashioned equipment, where a huge metal brace was screwed into my upper jaw for two months. (Both teeth were saved, but over the years, one of the teeth would gradually discolour and withdraw into my gums until I had a gap-toothed appearance. And, of course, this being England, no thought was given to the idea of rescuing the dental situation. In all of my photographs up until my early thirties, when I finally had my teeth fixed, I have this Mona Lisa, lips-closed smile.)

This event certainly happened at the right time – just six weeks before my personality change. But is it enough to explain it? I'd never believed so. I'd also supposed that the incident, where my dad had commented upon my skinny wrists, could have played a role. When I'd joined my new junior high school at the end of summer, wearing that huge metal brace, it could well have coincided with the period immediately after my dad's comment about my wrists, and this reinforcement might, because of my inordinate sensitivity, have caused me to believe I was tolerably hideous: not just an ugly skinny body, but also one bearing a mouth full of metal. But I'd still never felt, for some reason, that this was an explanation which fully resonated with me.

Broken Whole

But now I'd just recognized a third factor which was the key to it all. Our house had been right on the edge of two school districts, which meant that all of my former school friends had gone to a different school. Consequently, I knew nobody at all in the school, and since I was indeed not easy on the eyes with my braces, and awkward, skinny body, nobody wanted to be my friend. All that first year I had only one friend, the most unpopular girl in school (who was sexually assaulted and murdered one year later.)

This came to me now with a firm ring of truth: an explanation of why I went through grade school a pale shadow of my former self. I'd thought myself ugly, and so had others. But the reason this new realization hit me with so much force now, sitting at that restaurant on Santa Monica Boulevard after the cold-call at the modelling agency, was that I suddenly saw the life-long implications of that confluence of random circumstances. No sooner had the first insight struck, than the deep, undeniable certainty grew upon me that through those four years of friendlessness, I'd learned to think of myself as unlovable, unlikable, and uninteresting. And through the course of youth and young adulthood that deep self-hatred had settled into hidden places in my heart. On the surface, I'd recovered some of my gloss in college and grad school, but I never fully inhabited myself. Instead, in my mid-20s, the jealousy that had ravaged me during my relationship with Xavier began to exhume the self-loathing that had been laid down during grade school, sending me into a tail-spin of chronic fatigue and depression. And revisionistically, in my late thirties after I'd recovered fully from chronic fatigue, and had emerged from a decade as a hermit, I'd looked back at my life seeing only the loneliness, forgetting how easily I'd formed friendships in college and grad school.

All of a sudden, the entire path of my life, leading up to the crisis of the summer, was made clear to me. Just two split seconds in my life – two tiny pebbles dropped in the stream of life: my dad grabbing my wrists, and my slip in the bathroom. They could easily never have happened; or they could have happened at a time when I wasn't joining a school as a stranger. Without those two tiny moments occurring when they did, I might have led a completely different life; a life without decades of insecurity, chronic fatigue and depression, and ultimately, a huge manic episode, the latter being due, in part, to the belief that I'd finally come into my full inheritance of what I'd lost as a child.

Something that I'd always wondered about – what was the trauma that had triggered the chronic fatigue syndrome? – was now answered. It was, most likely, the accumulated layer of many hurts, most prominently amongst which was the rejection of my body by my dad in the incident with the skinny wrists.

I began to cry, sitting right there at the table in the restaurant. I started to weep, something I'd been doing a lot that summer. But this time the tears were of empathy: for the years of lost promise. I hadn't needed to have had so many dark and lonely years. I could have retained that glow I'd had as a seven-year-old and been somebody special without the burden of mania. It was ironic that I was uncovering this insight – something I'd always longed to understand – only due to the remaining manic brilliance lingering from my summer-long episode.

With tears still in my eyes, I ordered my food, and then returned to my writing. Despite my grief at those lost years, I was feeling thankful too: that I had at least forty more years left during which I could loosen myself from the strands that had bound me during my first forty years. And moreover, had I not taken the path that fate, chance or karma had determined to be mine, I'd never have met Ben.

I'd found the answer, at long last: those pebbles that had been dropped into the stream of my life in my eighth year. What remained to be understood is the answer I'd really been searching for throughout the summer of 2006. As I wrote my blog after the encounter at the modelling agency, I still felt that great things were in my future, now that my strengths were no longer held in check by depression. But the answer remained: what was the destination?

The Void, Paris, October

In October, Ben and I stayed in Paris for nine nights. I was feeling good: the mania was, I thought, gone; I'd accepted I was bipolar; I remained convinced that my oldest enemy, depression, was dead and buried; and I was grateful, above all else, for the positive effects of the changes wrought in the summer, and the complete loss of neuroses that had been with me since childhood. I remained full of life, vitality, energy and self-confidence; and expected to be like that the rest of my life. I didn't need to drink when we met friends at a bar, because the stage of conviviality and loose inhibitions which people use alcohol to reach, was now a constant for me. I knew I'd be returning to work full-time after our return from Paris, but was also looking forward to continuing with some of my ideas at the same time, *Club Karma* in particular.

Ben had been invited to lecture at the Pasteur Institute, and on the day of his presentation, I took the opportunity to spend a night in London visiting my family, seeing them for the first time since the crisis. On the night I got back, I received an email from Dean which shook me to the core, because it made me abruptly realize that the goal on which I'd pinned all of my hopes might actually be out of reach. There was a fatal flaw in my grand scheme for becoming a glamorous party-promoter in West Hollywood, and it was, in retrospect, a screamingly obvious flaw. Once more, the blinding light of manic thinking had obscured common sense, but Dean's email gave me a sudden moment of clarity. Several weeks earlier I'd made the decision to be completely open about my diagnosis of bipolar disorder. It was all over my blog, and while Dean didn't directly say it, his email made me realize that nobody would invest in a limelight-hogging business headed by a man who was mentally ill. (This latter perception was itself likely erroneous given I live in Hollywood.)

It came down to making a choice between continuing to be open about being bipolar or giving up my dream of being a party promoter. And for about twenty minutes that night I hovered on the edge, unwilling to face the fact that I'd have to give up such a gorgeous dream, but also facing the suddenly looming prospect of a return to depression brought on by shame – the shame I'd surely feel if I closeted my bipolar disorder. And sure enough, as my conclusions sank home, I felt the familiar thickening of the head that marked the return to depression after six months without it.

I felt idiotic that I hadn't foreseen that depression could return. Why hadn't I come to the obvious conclusion that bipolar disorder clearly implies two poles: manic, and depressive? Why hadn't my therapist or psychiatrist forewarned me when I claimed to them that I'd never be depressed again? As my heart and spirit sank with fear, I began to think of all the consequences. Which of my other dreams might I have to give up now that I'd seen how easily depression could return?

Wanting to be a party promoter was easy to understand. Who wouldn't understand that desire, particularly in West Hollywood, the home of some of the biggest gay dance events in the world? I'd grown immensely attracted to the idea. I knew I'd be good at it: I loved being around people, I was creative, I felt I could charm anybody, and I was well organized. Above all else, it appealed to the idea of making up for the decades of feeling *other than*: I felt that it would make me the sort of person everybody wanted to know. And I believed my idea of a gay club free of attitude was something new: that I could bring much needed Karma to West Hollywood. It would also, of course, get me out of debt – assuming I made a success of it.

Shame was the problem. The summer's crisis had resolved itself firstly through medication, but also, crucially, by burning away decades of shame, and self-hatred; a shame which had expressed itself physically through almost twenty years of chronic fatigue syndrome, and mentally through fifteen years of chronic depression.

As I'd learned through David, openness is the opposite of shame. That concept was the origin of my decision to be thoroughly open about my bipolar disorder: if I once let myself feel shame over it – like I had for my depression - I knew I'd end up mired in prolonged depression once again. In other words, if I stopped writing my blog so that my public persona could be hygienic enough to be a business man, a party promoter, I'd be giving into shame, and heading towards depression.

In our hotel room in Paris, as I thought things through while Ben showered, I felt horror sweeping over me; as if a pit was yawning open in front of me into which I might tip head-first. It's impossible to describe the sheer panic that welled up from my gut. In the space of twenty minutes I'd gone from knowing for sure that I'd be depression-free for life, to worrying that it had come back full-strength to destroy all the illusions about what I could accomplish; about who I actually was. How could I meet with people and marshal them into subscribing to my dreams if I felt, once again, so completely unsure about myself? I saw all my hopes vanishing to the horizon. With every second, in a nightmare reverse of the moment on the day of insanity when I'd had the customer service idea and had seen my life changing by the second, new consequences rendered themselves vividly in my consciousness: new friends who'd been attracted by the strength of my self-belief would see that it had all been a paper tiger; acquaintances who'd been drawn in by my plans would be disappointed and angry; I'd have to ignominiously re-emerge into the society of my friends as a depressed person, no longer sure of myself, embarrassed by my former loud claim that I was free of depression for life.

My therapist was out of reach in California for several days; I knew I was in an acute crisis, a crisis which, given what I'd put Ben through this summer, had to be kept to myself. And what should I choose to do: hold onto the – now seemingly impossible – dream of being a party-promoter; or continue to shun shame by writing openly about my diagnosis? Did I, in fact, have any choice?

The initial crisis resolved itself, later that afternoon, while I was writing at a corner café in the Latin quarter, looking out at the sidewalks, which glistened with rain and the lights reflecting from store windows. With deep sadness, I decided I had no choice but to continue with the blog, and let go of the club. I couldn't risk going into shame. Karma had been a wild ride, and I didn't put it to bed without tears.

There was also one further inevitable conclusion. I'd thought that the mania had passed, and that the remaining self-confidence was the "real me" left by the retreating wake of both depression and mania. Now it seemed that, until the crisis of confidence, I'd still been, in fact, manic. What if I had yet to discover the real me?

The rest of our stay in Paris proved a difficult challenge. I wrestled with the upsetting discovery that I could still experience depression. The key question for me became: what did this mean, apart from its implication for dropping Karma? Without my therapist being available, and scared of worrying Ben, I was left entirely on my own to assess this question. I hadn't yet read enough about bipolar disorder to know what was expected. I'd assumed that the medication I was taking would simply control my new ebullient personality from elevating into mania.

One of the greatest blessings of the manic period had been the deletion of almost all of the former neuroses that had antagonized my depression. But, one night, towards the end of our stay, I hit another moment of sudden, acute panic. Ben was out of the room on an errand, and the bottom dropped out of my heart, as I confronted, for the first time, the awful possibility that I'd made no progress at all; that I'd experienced no healing by going through the crisis with Ben. What if I was now the same person I was in April, before my manic episode? Would it all come back: the jealousy, the insecurities, the need to compete, the social discomfort, the vulnerability to being slighted or ignored, the fear of abandonment, the guy who was so depressed he was willing to sacrifice his sex life by taking Lexapro? Underneath me the ground dropped vertiginously into a yawning chasm, this time a vast void.

I panicked. What if all my grand conclusions about myself: that I had guts; that I no longer required physical validation; that I'd found my soul: what if these were just the detritus of the supernova that had gone off in my head this summer, a nebula now receding in the darkness? Had everything – absolutely everything – been ephemeral? How was I going to get through the rest of the trip? How was I even going to get through this evening, having dinner with Ben and Jean-Marc, our good friend? How could I tell Ben about this without imbuing him with as much fear as I felt?

While Ben was still out of our hotel room, I wrote in my private leather-bound journal – the same journal I'd bought at the end of the hellish week in Dallas:

> *It's been a devastating discovery these last two or three days, that I can still feel deep depression. I thought it was gone for good. For the moment, the strong, self-confident, care-free guy of the last six months has been completely eradicated. Knowing that I have to be social with Ben and Jean-Marc in a few minutes, I look at myself in the mirror and tell myself urgently, 'I'm still the same person I was a week ago.' But I see a disbelieving death's head in the mirror, a scarred soul whose inner darkness is written on his features. And what if the quite different person I saw a week ago in the mirror was not the real me? I think the kernel of shame is still inside me, and the realization that Karma might not work out has swept over the wall of my defenses, swamping the blazingly self-confident Keith of three days ago.*
>
> *I have to choose very carefully what I say to Ben, because everything feels so precarious. One*

moment I think I may be able to regain that strong sense of self; the next moment I'm literally trembling, on a roller-coaster of shame, about things I've recently promised or said about myself: things which now seem laughably unattainable in the light of departed self-confidence.

The truth is I'm scared; petrified. The magnificent future I'd erected in my mind's eye seems suddenly impossibly out of reach. Yet now, as Ben returns into the room, and smiles at me, I can't tell him a thing. How can I tell him that the bottom has dropped out of my life? I'm completely unprepared for this, and I'm finally not sure that even writing about it is helping.

Yet now I'm lying on the bed while Ben dresses for dinner; in ten minutes I may be past this temporary panic (as has already happened several times). That is how unstable the ground is right now. I'm breathtakingly scared, yet I have nobody to turn to, and must hide it all from Ben.

I didn't know whether I'd just refused to listen, had not heard what I'd been told, or had genuinely been left unprepared for the return of depression; but this sudden discovery was a terrible shock. Just when I thought I'd found stable ground, here was a new shift. And how far was the shift?

I was rescued, however, from the extremities of such despairing thoughts that very evening. My deepest worry had been that I was completely unchanged by my manic episode. But something showed me that I had indeed changed permanently; it allowed me to see that, scary though it was, what I was experiencing was the return of garden-variety organic depression, a natural down-swing as part of bipolar disorder.

We'd been to a bar with Jean-Marc, and there had been quite a few sexy men who'd noticed Ben. When we got home, Ben wanted to have sex. But I was taking my time, thinking about writing a blog, and how to express myself without tipping off Ben about how I was feeling. Ben said that if he'd known I was going to write, he would have just stayed at the bar.

It was thoughtless; in fact almost insulting – implying that if he'd stayed at the bar he could have had sex with one of the admiring strangers, and that that would have substituted for having sex with me. Of course, he didn't really mean it that way. For one thing, we're monogamous. But it's an exemplar of the sort of offhand, thoughtless comment of which he was occasionally capable, would have triggered a feeling of extreme hurt in the old, depressed Keith. Beyond a shadow of a doubt, that person would have sheltered this thoughtlessness in his heart, and stoked it, as if desiring the pain; as if deserving the thoughtless act. I'd have been aggrieved at Ben, and would have harboured that feeling until the next morning. And, of course, I'd have withheld sex.

But now, without even really thinking about it, I smiled at Ben. His comment said nothing about me. Ben was simply being thoughtless, out of momentary irritation. Whether he ultimately realized it himself or not, it was about him, not about me.

We were both tired, so I just told him to think about what he'd just said; in the morning he'd realize how thoughtless it was, and then I went back to thinking about my blog. But as Ben banged around bad temperedly in the bathroom, I looked up as I registered the lack of hurt to the slight he'd given me. It was very obvious to me that, even though I felt the organic depression, my sense of self wasn't damaged by what Ben had said. I wondered if, indeed, the months of manic fire had, as I'd originally thought, sought out the most deep-seated of my insecurities, and purged them.

Over the next few weeks, as I struggled with the new found depression, I saw many such incidents play themselves out, confirming my initial conclusions. Despite the return of depression, I wasn't right back where I'd been in April: I'd permanently dropped a whole ton of baggage.

Book V – Broken Whole
Broken? 2007

Although I now felt assured that a lot of my insecurities were gone for good, I still had to cope with the organic depression that had returned in Paris. I didn't yet know if shame and lack of joy would return also.

At first, I thought I'd try a new coping strategy by pretending the depression wasn't there. But there was still the issue of my blog. Writing breezily in the blog as if I wasn't depressed: what was the point of that? So I had to choose between not disclosing it, or being open – both to Ben and in my blog. But when I analyzed the problem, it seemed both routes led back to depression. It was a no-win scenario, on the surface, unless I could somehow cut the automatic link between shame and depression.

My first instinct was indeed to write about depression, but to do so in an engaging way. I didn't want every entry to sound like 'Oh, my God, I'm so depressed today.' So I wrote about what I was learning, and even tried to write metaphorically about my experience of rediscovering depression, using Churchill's "black dog" to describe the arc of my journey through depression and mania and back again.

> *I was low and weak. The black dog bided its time. I turned finally to face it, exposing my neck, and the creature leaped, sinking its teeth deep. My hands clawed at its head, and finally it let go its grip and bounded away.*

> *Those initial wounds were the worst, and I doubt they'll ever leave me.*

> *It was a few years until I saw the black dog again. This time I was more prepared, and I was able*

Broken Whole

to fight it off. But over the years, it would return again and again to stalk me. I never let it at my throat again; I sought constantly for new ways to fend it off, and even kill it.

Then something wonderful happened, and I assumed what I thought was my true form: that of a white dog, with blazing eyes, and fangs every bit as sharp as his. I remember now the deep blood satisfaction I felt as I tore at him for the first time, and the wild look of fear in his eyes as he retreated.

For a while, I thought he might return, and I kept watch. But weeks later, I heard tales that his carcass had been found in the hills, and I thought myself finally in the clear. It was as if a great cloud had been lifted.

So the shock was yet greater when he suddenly returned, gnawing this time at my vitals. For a few moments I thought he had won; that this was the final fight. My disguise was shredded. His prolonged absence had so disarmed me that I'd forgotten how to fight.

I was just able to free myself from his teeth, and I turned to face him. We circled each other, and I saw that it had become a standoff. In his absence, I now recognized I'd learned some new survival skills. I knew I couldn't kill him, but I could see in his eyes that he knew he couldn't kill me either.

Now his bites, when he comes at me from behind, still sting. Yet he cannot destroy me. The open skies I knew when I thought him dead; sure, they were an illusion; and I have to live with his angry maw again. But I'll try out new lines of attack. I will never let the black dog win.

It took me two weeks after Paris to be sure that joy could coexist – at least intermittently – with the organic depression. Before my summer-long manic episode, shame, my depressive mood disorder and the organic depression had all been hopelessly linked: three black holes bound together in tight orbits. Of course, once I'd been diagnosed as bipolar, I'd believed all three were gone for good, taking with them the root cause – a deep-seated self-dislike. When organic depression had returned in Paris, I'd expected the shame and lack of joy to return too, particularly since I had so many new things to be ashamed of now, most obviously my manic spending, the abandonment of my entrepreneurial endeavours, and the disappointment of friends.

But, in those early weeks after Paris I found myself simultaneously feeling the physical sensations of depression – heaviness in the head – while also feeling, at times, a sense of joi-de-vivre. It was a strange, new sensation, but not unwelcome. I even, for a while, slowly revived the idea of the club. But then I went through three weeks of utter blackness, probably triggered by being overly medicated against mania. After that, a new pattern emerged: no sooner would I come to a firm conclusion about my moods, than the subsequent weeks would prove me wrong. Mania and depression began chasing each other's tails. I had to accept that I couldn't yet trust my mental condition, and therefore couldn't risk disappoint people all over again. Bit by bit I dropped almost all of the plans I'd formed during my manic phase. I gave up the club idea for good this time, and then the customer service idea, which, now that the fog of mania had cleared, I could easily see was of dubious legality. And even though I was badly in debt, I also had to give up, under legal advice, the idea of winning damages by prosecuting the Omni Hotel and the LAPD. My lawyer told me that once the opponents dragged in my bipolar diagnosis, as they surely would, it would be a difficult case to win. Moreover, I couldn't put Ben through such unsavoury hell.

It took a long time for me to accommodate myself to the new symptoms of bipolar disorder, both psychological and physical. Chief amongst the latter remained a feeling that electricity was surging through my body culminating in a live terminal at the top of my head. I'd become physically clumsy too. Other sensations were so bizarre I couldn't even quite describe them: my feet would feel warm and tingling; I almost felt as if I could directly perceive the pulse beating in my neck; and when I turned my head there was the inward impression of my bones creaking in their sockets. I was scared of these physical phenomena, and sought self-medication to dampen them. Ben and I had discovered the new *Battlestar Galactica*, now in its third season. It became our thing – a sort of comforting refuge, during this period of recovery – to spend an hour or two each night watching the show on DVD from the beginning. It was towards the end of the day, when we'd be watching *Battlestar*, that the electricity in my head would reach its apex. I'd tell Ben to hit the pause button on the DVD player, claiming to want to go upstairs to "go to the bathroom", or "get some cheese", but in reality rushing straight for the vodka bottle in the freezer in order to quench the flames within. I stashed little bottles of vodka in various hiding places around the house in case I couldn't reach the bottle in the freezer without Ben seeing. (Ben will learn this for the first time when he reads this.)

And every few weeks, initially, I could clearly identify the return of some of the mental sequels of mania, in a milder form called hypomania, such as flight of thoughts, the almost uncontainable desire to connect with other people – principally strangers, and, more dangerously, the beckoning call to invest my time – if no longer my money, for I was broke – in pursuit of new ideas. These moods would return with slowly diminishing frequency, like a stone skipping on the surface of a lake, alternating with periods where depression would abruptly – in a matter of seconds – return like a huge dark wall obscuring the horizon.

Since there seemed to be no resting point between bipolar swings, I learned not to make pronouncements about the future. In the early summer of 2006, before I'd become verifiably manic, I'd grandly announced to my closest friends that depression had permanently departed from my life. I could not have been more wrong. And when I'd spent most of December back in the fog of depression, I'd written in my blog that I would probably stop writing, because I didn't want to just write about depression. Verifiably wrong again. So, no more pronouncements, I swore. I acknowledged that I was heading into uncharted territory.

Of the creative pursuits begun under mania, all that remained was my book, which I was still working on. But having dropped so many other things so quickly, I now felt like the ultimate dilettante. And to make matters worse, I had to live with decisions I'd made under the assumption that I would never again go into depression. Ever since I'd moved to Los Angeles, my employers had wanted me to work at home so that they could shut down their expensive office in Century City in which I was then the sole employee. But I'd resisted, knowing that working at home, in our house in a quiet part of the Hollywood Hills, wouldn't be good for my depression. However, there was a long period after my diagnosis of bipolar disorder during which I'd experienced no depression at all, and I'd assumed, wrongly, that I'd now be fine working at home. So now, once the depression had returned, I was saddled with long days at home, alone in a house where you walked out of the door to experience almost complete silence.

Things at home were made worse by the lack of work for many months after I returned from disability. I remained unsure about how I was perceived at work. I'd not hear from my boss for weeks at a stretch, and wondered if I was being withheld from projects because of doubt about my manageability and efficacy. I found out weeks after the fact that I'd been the only person in my division not invited to headquarters for a pow-wow where new positions were offered up as promotions. Even if work were to come, I had my own doubts to deal with. I was still subject to moments of cognitive confusion where my mind would feel like syrup, and I wondered how I'd fare under the pressure of challenging work in front of other people.

The expected life-span of people with bipolar disorder is identifiably shorter than for the general population. I take this to be due not directly from the physical effects of the disease, but a consequence, instead, of manic-fuelled risk-taking and impaired decision-making resulting in death or injury, and self-medication for depression and mania in the form of drugs and alcohol. For a while, I'd been scared that *I* was in danger of making alcohol a part of my daily life. That had not happened, but I did understand intimately the risks of death or injury due to a fogged mind. One day, two helicopters roared very loudly over the top of our house, heading towards a fire across the valley from us, on the backside of the hill on which the Hollywood sign was mounted. Not recognizing the sudden racket, I'd rushed out of the glass doors onto our balcony. Or at least that was the intention. Unfortunately, the glass door was actually shut. It was made of untempered glass, as I discovered when I tried to run through it: it shattered, leaving a two foot jagged shard in the door frame, exactly at kidney level. It was easy to imagine Ben coming home to find me impaled upon it, a pool of blood at my feet. I'd been saved by my prominent nose, which alone had touched the glass.

I was still taking Xanax, for sleep, along with a colourful selection of mood-stabilizers and anti-depressants, and it suddenly occurred to me, on a visit to my psychiatrist, that perhaps some of the mind confusion and abnormal physical symptoms – as puzzling to my psychiatrist as they were to me – could be a reaction to medication. She reduced my dosage of Depakote, which indeed had, as a side-effect, confusion and other cognitive impairments, and switched me from Xanax to Klonopin, which has a longer half-life, setting me on a plan to gradually wean me entirely of anti-anxiety medication. After my session, I looked up online the list of withdrawal symptoms experienced at the end of a day, almost twenty-four hours after taking your last Xanax, and there, in print, were some of the exact sensations I'd experienced. In fact, I'd been spared some of the truly grisly ones, such as the sense that your teeth are rotating in their sockets.

I finally got a new work project, and had to stay in New Jersey, just outside of Manhattan, for three weeks, away from Ben for the first time since the crisis. The first day on the job was the worst. When I pulled my laptop out of my brief case, in front of a colleague, it came out dripping wet. I've never been so glad that my affinity is for vodka – clean and odourless – instead of something like tequila, since my co-workers seemed to accept that it was a water bottle that had spilled in my bag, instead of my emergency supply of self-medication. I rushed my laptop and briefcase to the men's room, where I scooped up the remaining vodka, and slurped it from my hands to still the electricity now surging through my head again, playing havoc with my mental processing skills. Before going back into the office, I tried to see how my laptop responded to electricity, and fired it up. Due to an earlier problem with my work laptop, it was my own heavily tricked out Sony Vaio, bought during the first weeks of mania. It was completely fried. Karma had come full circle.

Somehow, though, I survived those three weeks, and did good work, and I concluded, with relief, that I could still hack it. But I could hardly continue to rely upon alcohol to mediate my moods and physical symptoms. I experimented with playing with changing the dosages of my medications, as my level of depression or hypomania waxed and waned, and tried to apply either techniques such as mindfulness, and my own – self-discovered at need – form of meditation. But, more than anything, I began to rely on a careful choice of activity as a self regulator. I'd discovered early on that there were things that could both swiftly propel me into hypomania, as well as trigger the physical sensations I dreaded. These included passionate conversation, pushing heavy weights at the gym, intellectual discoveries, and even bathing myself in the all-surrounding finale of a Mahler symphony in my car. Almost any activity could do it, if it engaged the mind, or my senses, and was sustained long enough. In the midst of a game of cards with Ben and Stephane, for instance, in Palm Springs, my competitive instinct kicked in, and before long I had to "go to the bathroom" – my new euphemism for the consumption of vodka.

In view of the catalogue of incidents which had led me to be arrested, I also had to learn to avoid confrontation – to still the urge to point out and attempt to rectify wrongs. This was one of the most difficult challenges: it felt like I was cutting off my left thumb in curtailing a part of my personality that I thought of not only as a strength, but as a fundamental part of my selfhood. I had an early opportunity to put into action this new practice of letting things go. I was heading up through the winding, hilly streets above West Hollywood to see my therapist, and rounded the corner to find the road blocked by a hulking Mercedes SUV. I couldn't get past him, because just as I stopped behind the SUV, a guy coming in the other direction in a vintage Porsche convertible pulled up in the other lane directly abreast of the SUV. The driver got out, retrieved something from the SUV, which was obviously his, and saw, apparently, no problem in my just sitting there waiting for him. It was the sort of self entitled, LA behaviour that would have formerly made my blood boil. But I didn't say anything, breathed a few mantras in my head, and was rewarded with a healthy dose of Schadenfreude. As he returned to his convertible, smoke started coming out of the engine. He rolled it into his driveway, thus clearing the road, just in time for flames to start shooting out of the back of his car (I kid you not). I hit the gas and shot up the hill in case his car exploded. I'd mention karma here if it weren't for my suspicious that you're probably growing tired of the subject.

Since I'd discovered that there were activities that might promote hypomania, I'd begun to toy with them as an antidote to depression. I was beginning to feel that my mood swings were manageable, although I also asked myself the question whether it wasn't a little vainglorious and perhaps ... manic ... to believe I could control my own mania. And how much of a good mood was too much? Despite the risks, if I was feeling oppressed by the relentless weight of depression, I'd try to engage myself in an activity that I knew could stimulate my thinking and – with the understood danger of triggering hypomania – raise my mood. But the boundary between feeling good in a good way, and feeling good in a way that overshot hypomania right into its more virulent form, mania, was very narrow. I liked to think that I could just pry open the lid of the box I'd placed around my mania for enough time to steal a few gleams of supernova light. But I knew that the restrained light could erupt from its captivity, and scorch everything in its path, if I didn't act quickly enough.

The hardest days were those where I could feel both the symptoms of depression and hypomania on the same day; even at the same time. Then, it seemed, there was nothing I could do about it, since going too far in either direction would be self-destructive. I was trying to stay carefully balanced on an extremely narrow surfboard atop the bipolar wave. Only time would tell if my approaches were workable in the long run. I shared what I was doing with Ben, my psychiatrist and my therapist, and everybody seemed to be on board with it (on the narrow, bipolar surfboard, so to speak.)

A frequent part of the narrative of the lives of people with bipolar disorder is the willful abandonment of medication, particularly amongst those with a strong creative urge. Mania feels incredible. It can easily become addictive, fuelling bouts of intensive creativity while dispelling the greyness of life lived under the ever-present threat of depression. There is no doubt that I deeply missed my manic creativity, and the almost superhuman charge that mania had added to my life. The quality of my writing seemed a shadow of what it had been under mania. (At least it was less grandiose.) And I missed those days of dashing around the West Side of LA in my Land-Rover, hot-pink cell-phone perpetually at my ear, feeling I was cutting a figure. Now, if I saw people I'd got to know while I was manic, I'd either avoid them, or try to keep contact to a minimum. In return, they'd no doubt wonder what had happened to the hypercharged person I'd been during the summer. I was aware of this, and experienced, as I'd predicted, fresh shame. It was a letdown to once more feel so ... normal.

Now, if I wasn't busy on project work, I'd spend my day at Starbucks working on my book, occasionally stealing envious glances at other people engaged in deep discussion of a film project, or on the phone to their producer, remembering my own days of self-important busy work. In contrast with the people I enviously regarded, I was sitting alone, unrecognized, paralyzed by debt, struggling to structure a day that could loom with the empty shadow cast by depression.

It would have been so easy to secretly stop taking my medication. Yet I was never tempted to do so – not even once. I'd seen the devil within; had beheld the destruction it had caused in my relationships, not to mention my pocketbook, and knew that the good things that come with mania were not worth the risk of self-destruction. I felt some embitterment, however, that I could never allow myself to access those parts of that luminous being held enslaved by medication that were the most appealing and positive – that I couldn't, in effect, afford to be fully myself.

Whole, 2009

The story told in this book has been, in some ways, that of the search for self. During my late teens and early twenties, I'd regularly say to myself in the privacy of my mind that I didn't know who I was. My real self had been submerged by shyness, self-consciousness and a fear of being judged. Now that the vast wave that had swamped the summer of my forty-first year had receded, what remained in its wake? It felt like I was facing anew the same questions I'd started out with. Which of my various selves was the real one? Would I make anything of my life? I couldn't say I really knew the answers to those questions. My future, obviously, had yet to be written.

Certainly, things had changed for me: I'd now seen the extremes within. I knew that I had the capacity to be somebody much larger than I'd ever expected. Yet was that person the real me? Even three years on, I wasn't sure where the true point of stability lay. Was there – for me at least – any such thing as a real self? I envied people their ability not only to say, this is the real me, right now, but also to be so unaware that such identity problems existed that they never even asked themselves such questions.

In the months after the manic self had been absorbed, I'd been tantalized by the thoughts of what that person could achieve. But now I knew, from experience, that I couldn't afford to let myself completely inhabit the person I wanted to be, because that person was a danger to himself and others. Wasn't it enough that I was where I was? I'd long since learned to accept, guided by David, that I *had* made a success of my life. Although I had a serious mental illness, I was otherwise robustly healthy; I was singularly lucky in both my family and friends; I lived in a house in the Hollywood Hills with two dogs; had the sort of relationship with Ben – a very desirable man – which I'd have never thought possible of myself; had a well-paid job, which I enjoyed and which challenged me; and had the time to pursue enjoyable, creative and intellectually fulfilling pastimes. I recognized that I was a very fortunate man, and also that I'd made some of my own luck by not surrendering to the depression and chronic fatigue of my thirties. But I didn't seem to have the sort of temperament which would ever let me lay aside, completely, the questions about identity; nor did I feel I was capable of putting to rest the feeling that I had to make some kind of special mark on life.

In the days when it became increasingly likely that my book would be published, it slowly dawned on me that I'd achieved something I'd thought about since my early twenties in writing a book and having it published. The more I thought about it, the more I realized that I'd come full circle. It had been the dramatic change from being a seven-year old kid with big dreams and a sunny disposition, to being, just a few weeks later, an isolated, lonely boy, which had laid the seeds of the depression that would hit me in my twenties. And it's unlikely I'd have been propelled into mania had I not been coming from a background of depression (after all, it was an anti-depressant that had been one of the two villains responsible for triggering mania.) During that crazy summer of 2006, it had seemed that I was going to achieve much more than I'd ever expected of myself. I'd known I was going to be somebody. But, in October, when I'd crashed, you could say that personal history repeated itself as all of my new dreams floated away on the backwash of returning depression. But here was the full-circle: I'd been inspired with material to finally write and finish a book. Now the question was, did writing a book which had originated during the period where I'd once again been robbed me of my dreams – the book you're reading right now – represent that special thing I'd expected to do with my life, that special mark?

It didn't seem this way at first. When I'd begun to write the book in the fall of 2006, I could not have appreciated how hard it would be to get people to read it, let alone consider it for publication. The subject matter was too traumatic for my close friends and family to read, at least initially. Strangers, meanwhile, would read half way through the first chapter, and put it aside, fearing I was still genuinely crazy. (Or perhaps they'd reach the part where I impersonated the Anti-Christ in jail, and fling the book across the room with disbelief.) This raised the question, again, of the boundaries between sanity and normality. I could concede that if I was writing about crazy things, how could an uninformed person know that I was in my right mind when writing the book? People might wonder if the whole thing was the product of a delusional mind.

The truth was that I did start writing this book before I was fully recovered. And just as there were sections that had been written in the spring of 2007, in the months after the shocking discovery, in Paris, that I could still experience denaturizing depression, there were also sections written while I was hypomanic. Was the latter writing invalidated by my state of mind? Was it any less me? How about the depressive part? Surely you couldn't say that the depressive writing was valid if the manic wasn't? What about other writers? Should we only take their writing seriously if we knew it was written whilst the author was in an equable mood?

I could understand people being wary of my writing. After all, when I'd been manic, I'd convinced people of my great plans. They'd had no idea I was manic. You don't automatically assume that people are crazy; you tend to take them at face value. If I'd appeared creative, ambitious, persuasive and energetic, it seemed reasonable to assume that to be my nature. In fact, I'd been weaving a tissue of unreality. It was ironic that the only time I'd been believed – at least by people who didn't know me – had been when *I really had been* crazy. And truly the most painful aspect of that time had been the lack of belief in my ideas from friends and family, which had left me feeling extremely betrayed. Since then, though, I'd gained the perspective to look back and wonder why Ben and my friends didn't entirely deserted me.

Broken Whole

Most people think of sanity as being such a concrete thing: you either have it or you don't, and there's no in between. But people who've been through experiences like mine know not only that sanity rests on shifting sand - you don't know where to stand in order to experience stability, but that there is really no such thing as the true self.

A person might be tempted to think of somebody with mental illness as somehow broken. Certainly, your own perspective can be coloured by others' reactions. Unlike an obviously physical illness, people – even your closest intimates – feel as if they have to behave differently towards you if you have a mental illness, and this can leave you feeling a little ... damaged, or even broken. Although the phrase *broken whole* had come to me at the culmination of the worst night in my life, while scribbling eighty pages through a long sleepless night in the psych ER lock-up, as a description of a world where complexity, with its step-brother chaos, were winning the battle of wholeness and purity, it came to have a multiplicity of meanings for me. It represented a feeling that I'd survived that night of hell despite what I had seen, at the time, as the LAPD's effort to break me. And, although I hadn't known then that I was bipolar, you could hardly think of two more polar opposite words than *broken* and *whole*.

Postscript
Thanksgiving, November, 2009

Surprisingly, it was only the other day, a week before sending the final version of this manuscript to the publisher, that the true, deep meaning of *broken whole* sunk home to me. The illness – bipolar disorder – that some might say causes me to be broken, is contained within the same person as the more luminous being I now know I have the capacity to be. I am whole in the sense that both sides – polar opposites – lie within me.

As I sit here on the day after Thanksgiving, at Starbucks, in Westwood, near the UCLA campus, all seems much as it was at the beginning of 2006, almost as if the whole thing never happened. I cycled into a new depression in June, and, although I know for a fact that it *will* come to an end when it wants to, the nagging voice inside can't help but ask *What if it doesn't?* Unlike unipolar depression, the depressive cycle of bipolar disorder is rarely amenable to conventional medical treatment, even though it feels to me exactly the same as the intermittent depression I became acquainted with in my late twenties. It would be easy to conclude that I'm in the same space – if you'll forgive the California phrasing – I was in four years ago. Yet if I look inside, I can see the changes wrought by both the months of tempest, the slow recovery, and the three years of coming to terms with living with bipolar disorder: the awakenings of spirituality, something I've long scorned; a move from relying on others' perceptions of my physical appearance to bolster my own self-esteem; knowledge that I can stand up for myself or others at need; and the discovery – perhaps the best possible outcome of the experience – that my depression can no longer be easily triggered by shame, conflict, and the other neuroses that were burned away in the fire of mania. The depressions I experience now are almost completely divorced

Broken Whole

from externalities: they are imposed by a neurological disease, whose depressive cycle is all but untreatable. I know that I'm *not* the same person I was four years ago, all appearances to the contrary. It's as if the experience that forms the core of this book broke everything apart into its constituent elements, and reassembled them into something new, which looks superficially much like the old, but is somehow more integrated ... more whole.

Acknowledgements

I'd like to thank my siblings Kirstie, Neil, and Sally: it turns out they're not brats after all; who knew? I'd like to be breezy, and avoid embarrassing them with the sort of sentiment we were all raised not to express, but, in all honesty, I was touched by their sensitivity and support both during and after the crisis, and it reminded me how lucky I am to have had such a great family. I was extraordinarily fortunate in my choice of parents, and I wish I could take credit for it. Although it took me many years to appreciate it fully, the example of my parents' love for one another and their children, as well as their common-sense, good British values, put in place a foundation in my own life that allows me to think of myself as a decent person too.

Many friends have contributed, some without knowing it, and of these, I'd like to particularly mention my closest Los Angeles friends, Dean, of course, Lam, Bill & Stephane, Tom & Marvin, and Andy & Bryan; and, in San Francisco, Cecilia, Randy & Kean, Mike, Tony, Terry and Brett as well as other dear further-flung friends, Shaun, Jean-Marc, Heike, John-Paul, and, in New York, Phoenix and Chris. In West Hollywood, the members of wonderful gang are too numerous and individually delightful to name or single out. The way they all accepted me without judgement, even though I was clearly not quite all there, will always be a touching memory. As with many gay men, our friends have become our family.

Thanks to Ina Hillebrandt, who gave great me direction for the book when I came to a thudding halt, as well as the staff of Starbucks store #633 on Santa Monica Blvd and Westmount in West Hollywood for providing such a welcoming space in which to write. And, although he didn't intend it, Father Tony of the Farmboyz spurred me to finally create a version of the book about which I felt comfortable enough to start contacting agents and publishers.

I can't fail to forget to thank the kindness and care of Dr. David Epstein, Gabi Deak, Dr. Jon Kaiser, Dr. Bernard Bierman, and, in particular, Paul Kundinger MFT, our couples counsellor, without whom it's unlikely we'd have made it through the crisis as a couple. And the people at the San Francisco office of the company I work for were a great help and support for Ben when I was in the psychiatric system, in particular Joy and Hunter.

The list of people to whom I owe apologies for my behaviour when I went off the rails is extensive, and, regrettably, some of them I don't know by name, such as the people at the Mexican restaurant from whom I stole a bottle of tequila, and the guy at 7/11 on whose counter I poured said bottle of tequila. Of those I do know, I'd like to apologize to Karta, to Wes and Myles of the Power Zone, and to Daryl K. Roach.

To Dean Whitehead, both Ben and I owe a sincere debt of gratitude. He dropped everything and went way beyond the demands of friendship on the night I was arrested. And his kindness, friendship and support have been pillars of my life for most of my five years in Los Angeles.

About Ben, there's not much more I can say. If this book doesn't convey his strength, and sheer humanity, then it's doubtful anything I ever write could do so. It says a lot about Ben that this is not even the first book to be dedicated to him. His best friend, Joe Lee, wrote the first openly gay novel published in Singapore, *Peculiar Chris*, and included Ben prominently in the dedications, saying "thanks for the courage." I don't think I ever, in my life, expected to find a soul mate. I was never completely convinced that such a thing existed. But Ben has proven me wrong, and I feel I'm the luckiest man in the world.

www.ingramcontent.com/pod-product-compliance
Ingram Content Group UK Ltd.
Pitfield, Milton Keynes, MK11 3LW, UK
UKHW041410180426
11947UKWH00007B/51